DO THIS!
NOT THAT!

DO THIS!

NOT THAT!

The Ultimate Handbook of Counterintuitive Parenting

Anna Glas
Åse Teiner

Translated by Malou Fickling

Skyhorse Publishing

Skyhorse Publishing books may be purchased in bulk at special discounts for sales promotion, corporate gifts, fund-raising, or educational purposes. Special editions can also be created to specifications. For details, contact the Special Sales Department, Skyhorse Publishing, 307 West 36th Street, 11th Floor, New York, NY 10018 or info@skyhorsepublishing.com.

Skyhorse® and Skyhorse Publishing® are registered trademarks of Skyhorse Publishing, Inc.®, a Delaware corporation.

www.skyhorsepublishing.com

10 9 8 7 6 5 4 3 2 1

Library of Congress Cataloging-in-Publication Data is available on file.

ISBN: 978-1-62087-780-7

Printed in the United States of America.

Contents

Introduction

Our goal is to encourage parents to think for themselves, believe in themselves, and do what they feel is best for them, their children, and families—regardless of what others may think. This is how we came up with the idea for *Do This! Not That!* Silly thoughts and contrary thinking invite creativity and fresh ideas. Whenever we talk to new parents, we encourage them to think in new ways: different, bigger, smaller . . . whatever is needed. It's easy to get stuck in the same patterns of thought, which often means that we have closed the door to creativity. And we need to be creative and resourceful as parents. We are constantly put in situations that we need to deal with and relate to.

We strongly emphasize the importance of having fun as parents. Parenting should be fun, and we figure that what each parent is doing probably works for them. We are, therefore, not experts with advice for "lost parents." We assume that everyone has common sense and that all of us are qualified to be parents to our own children.

We want you to feel cheerful when reading this book. It encourages the use of common sense and all we want to prove is that thinking and behaving unconventionally is courageous, fun, and cool. We are not claiming that our way of thinking is the best, or even any good. It's just that things usually turn out well when we think in new ways.

And it's usually quite amusing!

This book includes stories from parents who decided to use contrary thinking when trying to solve the common problems of raising kids. But what's unconventional for me might not be for you. Your parenting is about doing what's contrary in your family. What's a 180-degree turn for you? But, which way you choose to rotate your compass is your choice.

Contrary thinking can at times seem completely twisted and actually a little scary. Imagine you're dealing with a child who refuses to put their coat on every morning. You get angry, worked up, sweaty, and tired; but what would happen if you just gave up and did nothing . . . or if you decided to stay ridiculously positive? Start by thinking "180 degrees" and your actual actions might end up being somewhere in the 90-degree range as a consequence of that thought. You are the only one who knows, or at least has an idea of, what's suitable in your home. When doing something differently, you'll experience something new. You've started from scratch, and that's a start. You will begin to see new solutions that were not apparent to you before.

It's common for parents to think that they have to resolve their parenting issues on their own. Many parents that we meet do this and so do we. It's always a good idea to discuss parenting with others, because if we only think in terms of solving one problem with our child we rarely resolve the bigger issues. Many of the problems we face as parents can't be solved, so why should we waste our energy?

Perhaps it comes down to handling situations as they arise rather than solving the bigger problem. We live in a society that is highly focused on solving problems. But if we apply that thinking to our parenting, it can become overwhelming. Solving one problem can often lead to having another. For example, nagging: How do we stop doing it? It seems that nagging and repeating everything are part of a parent's job description, but there must be a large number of parents who are sick of it. Sometimes nagging is necessary, but we can certainly find ways to deal with a predicament in other ways—maybe we can choose not to be bothered as much by something or make the best of the situation. It's more about tricking the mind, and if we, as parents, simply accept the fact that we need to nag, something changes in our approach. Many parents we've met have started thinking like this and feel relief because of it; it's one less battle. And when you talk to other parents who are going through the same battles, you realize that you're not alone. You might not be able to completely stop nagging, but you'll know how to manage a particular situation!

Let's continue looking at a parent's job description. For some strange reason, it's implied that all parents need to follow the same set of rules. These rules can be found in parenting literature or brochures that we receive when we are pregnant. They can also be declared by "parenting experts" we see on TV, or by friends, our parents, and neighbors. They provide a template for more obvious ways of dealing with problems.

What about the parts that aren't as obvious? Do we create our own templates for how we "should" be as parents? What are they based on? Are they of any use to us? Yes, maybe they are, and maybe the expert advice is of use too—sometimes. Difficulties and confusion arise at times when advice that "should" work doesn't. When I'm faced with a situation I can't handle as a parent, I often clutch at a piece of straw, a new way of doing something. But I often end up with a whole bale of hay on my head—dropped from above! We need to choose the straw, and the choice needs to be based on who I am, who my child is, whom I share my parenting job with, and in what way things work in our family. What works for one parent might not work at all for me. On this basis, we need to reflect on our very own, unique job description as a parent. What aspects do I need to pay attention to, what do I need to contemplate? I am the expert of my children and my situation. What does my job description look like? What help or what support do I want?

Is it possible to write a parenting book without mentioning the parent's role? It probably is, but let's think about it for a bit. The word itself is interesting. Do we play a role when we're with our children? What does that role entail? The answer is probably different for each one of us. The widespread image of the parenting role has certainly changed a lot in the last hundred years. Regardless of what has influenced it—the church, social movements, families, public radio, medicine, education—the approach is that we as parents must educate our children so that they function in the society they live in. A parent's role today is all about choosing for yourself and deciding what is the best for you and your children—in theory. That's easier in theory than in practice though, and we end up stuck in a gap between theory—thinking that we are free to do as we want—and in practice, which is often influenced by old habits and values. By becoming aware of how we think and what we actually do, we can make a decision to change.

Let's imagine that we are going to play the role of a parent. Who am I in the company of my child? What if you're only a human being? We have spoken to many parents who have told us how they "stepped out of the parental role" in order to handle a situation. This entailed leaving behind the "almighty" and "powerful" preconceptions, and, instead, revealing feelings, failing and trying again, horsing around and having fun, feeling a certain way about something one day and then feeling a different way another day—and they discovered the impact these new emotions had was so much greater.

We need to be aware of what we do and our way of thinking, and sometimes we need to review and analyze our parenting. We might look at what we've tried in the past and discover that it wasn't appropriate. What's done is done and we did what we thought was best in that moment. Let's move on. Then we can start thinking in new ways and do it with love and respect for ourselves. As a parent, it's easy to judge ourselves, and often those who talk about their unconventional methods feel the need to explain or make excuses for themselves. We want unconventional parents to be proud! They have started to become aware, reexamined the problem, and found a new (if slightly crazy) solution, and they've come far enough to take action. That's great! We envision that in the near future, there will be a swarm of unconventional parents proudly standing up for their cause. This is the way we do it and it works!

We can still continue comparing our pregnancies, births, the progress of our children, and our parenting skills with other parents, because we need to see the similarities and differences and find common ground. We need to reflect upon our parenting methods by seeing how others handle things, but some parents try to seem perfect and don't delve into the real problems they are dealing with. We, as parents, can and should help each other. We don't have to cope with everything on our own. One way could be to actually talk about our smallness, and share our difficulties and troubles with others. Another way is to be brave and stand up for our methods regardless of others' reactions. A third is to celebrate and encourage other parents who do what they believe in. When someone asks us a question, we should feel like we are being asked and not questioned.

In order to do the contrary, we need to be spontaneous and flexible. This is easier to do if you know what your limits and boundaries are as a parent, but it also depends on how you want to "shape" your children. The size of the surface varies for all of us. When we know the boundaries, we can move around freely in that space.

We need to be comfortable with the fact that we don't always know what the outcome will be. It might not turn out well at all . . . or it will turn out perfectly . . . or at least good enough.

We have to be able to deal with setbacks. They can be fun!

We also need to be able to handle success.

We may have to "kill our darlings." There is comfort in doing the same things over and over again, even when it no longer benefits us.

We may need to ask ourselves questions such as: How bad could it be? What's the worst that could happen? What's the best thing that could happen?

Sometimes, we need to do things that haven't been done previously. The brave have to lead the way, to help those who follow.

We may need support, guidance, and a pat on the back.

We need to prepare ourselves for lots of fun!

To conclude the introduction, we want to emphasize the benefits of doing things contrary to traditional methods. Contrary action cures perfectionism. We don't have to stress out about always being perfect. We can be lazy, we can be rebellious, and we can go our very own way.

Being unconventional increases our self-esteem and self-confidence. We have the courage to think in new ways, do new things, and change our behavior. We trust our ability to handle situations. We learn to like ourselves, regardless of success or failure. We can be less pristine around our children, others, and ourselves.

Contrary thinking also becomes a way for our children to deal with situations. Think of how it will benefit them!

Unconventionality is creating something new, and there is an intrinsic value in this, whether it makes life more fun, easy, or no different at all. We are one step closer to something better, or at least one step away from what we were unhappy with.

Do This! Not That! will give you some straws that you can pick up if you want and need to. See it as a bunch that you can use to make your own wreath or bouquet. We are confident that you are the best parent for your child and that you will make loving choices based on the details and the whole picture. Most times you'll be able to do it without a problem, but it's going to be challenging sometimes too—and that's okay!

Anna Glas & Åse Teiner

Growing as an adult

To become a parent is to grow as a person. After your first child is born you will do a crazy amount of growing, which may feel strange, different, and energy-consuming, but sometimes, it might feel completely opposite. It obviously depends on who you are, what kind of life you led previously, and what expectations you have. There are few things in life that drastically alter your existence as much as becoming a parent. Once the child is born, it's just there. You're a parent, period. But somehow, most people are able to handle becoming a parent. It's great, amazing, and admirable! Sure, people have been giving birth since forever, but it actually says a lot about our capacity as human beings.

You go from focusing on yourself and other things to now having to focus on your child above all else. If you can, don't let it go to your head! But while you are taking care of your child and yourself, you also have to handle everything that continues going on around you.

Many parents express just how difficult and tiring it is to sort out all the information about parenting. One mom told us: "Everyone complains about all the information that surrounds us in today's society. Wait until you have kids! Once you have a kid, it only increases, and it takes a lot of energy for me to organize all the information I receive about how I should take care of my child." When we started talking to her about common sense, she shrugged with annoyance and then exclaimed with a slightly hopeless tone: "I had common sense before I had children, but it sort of disappeared—it's a luxury." We have thought a lot about what that mother said. Sure, she was being humorous and said it with a twinkle in her eye, but what if there are more parents who think like this—they think that common sense was something they once had, that had disappeared and then reappeared as a type of luxury? It is nice to see common sense as a luxury, though, a luxury that we all have and actually could use. People will definitely grow when making use of that luxury, especially parents who are in great need of common sense.

We believe that one of the reasons that common sense is so difficult to use is because everyone feels the need to give advice to parents on how they should act and what they should do. Nowadays parents are hot prey. We want the very best for our children, but do we have the courage to take a chance and assume that common sense will lead us in the right direction? We could play it safe and choose the certain before the uncertain, so that we don't have to risk what's most precious to us—our kids. But who decides what we can and cannot do as parents? If you were to ask that question to parents, the majority would answer: "We do!" If we play with the idea that we are free to decide for ourselves, we would more easily be able to "indulge" ourselves in common sense. The road between theory and practice is sometimes frustratingly long. Or, you can reflect on what common sense consists of.

We believe that common sense is based on intuition, as well as experience, and that this is unique for each person—your common sense is yours alone. Which brings us to the next question: How much parenting experience do we have when it becomes our turn? Well, we may have none or we may have plenty. Looking back in time, people were often younger when they became parents. Information about parenting wasn't as widespread. Children were not as planned as they are today. This probably meant that people dealt with things in the moment—thinking on their feet, shooting from the hip. Many were also responsible for taking care of younger siblings and, therefore, had the experience and practical knowledge that they could use as a starting point when they became parents. Whether the past was better or worse is of less importance, since we are alive now, but it might serve as an explanation to make us understand something of use to us.

Parenting trends change. Nowadays we feel that the trend is to think for yourself and create your own system for your family, with society's rules in the background. Anything is normal!

This is where problems arise. While we must think for ourselves, often quickly, there is so much information, so much to think about. We're used to being told how we should do things, and now we are listening to how we could do things. There are thousands of theoretical outlines and methods we can use to solve our problems, find self-realization, and make decent people out of our children. Parents today are great at taking in information, but how well do we evaluate it all? It takes time to assess everything, just like the mother earlier in the book noted. That energy could instead be put toward "just being a parent." That mother became angry after a while and that gave her a lot of much-needed energy and high spirits. When other parents feel uncertain, however, it drains their energy. We are the most energized when we feel confident as parents. This is when we can grow. Feeling confident doesn't mean that we always know what we should do with our children and that we are never worried. Anxiety and uncertainty are feelings we can't escape as parents, or in life in general for that matter, and that certainly makes us human beings. But it doesn't necessarily have to come all at once. It's better when these feelings of anxiety come in little doses every once in a while.

As the "teachers" we are, we like working with the idea of the *knowledge stairs*. They have created security, insight, and growth for us, as well as for the parents we've talked to.

To explain what the knowledge stairs are, we'll give you an example. Let's take something as simple as diapering. You are expecting your first child and are currently on the *unconscious ignorance* step when it comes to this feat. You might have never changed a diaper, and expectant parents usually don't think about changing diapers—there are other things that are much more important. You are unaware of your ignorance of diaper changing; it's something that you don't reflect on whatsoever. On this step there is peace and quiet, but you aren't learning anything new either. And then suddenly, you're at the maternity ward and you're faced with a diaper full of brown, sticky goo. Without noticing it, you have taken a step up the ladder and landed on the *conscious ignorance* step. What do you do? Penis up, down, or

15

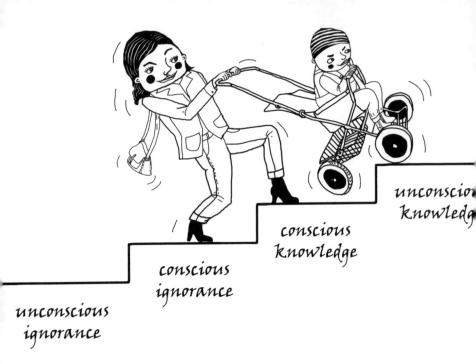

unconscious
knowledge

conscious
knowledge

conscious
ignorance

unconscious
ignorance

sideways? Which sides should be lifted? Soap *and* water, *just* water, or hand disinfectant (yes, sometimes it's really confusing)? Maybe you start doing it the way you think is best, or you ask for help, and surely it will all be fine in the end. Now you know how to change your baby's diaper and have, therefore, reached the happy, *conscious knowledge* step. This is great! You're a genius at diapering!

Next, you come home and you have to listen to "when you were little, we always used wipes made out of foam rubber—they were so easy to rinse out—but of course, you don't have running water next to your changing table . . ." or, "we think the ones made out of paper are the best, the bottom doesn't get as red and irritated," or, "the small washable cloths that can be reused are the best—we need to think a little about the environment, too." And there you are, leaving the maternity ward with a bag filled with practical ready-to-use wipes—perfect for those who mounted the changing table to the bedroom wall, with no direct connection to water. . . . This is when we must stand firmly on the *conscious knowledge* step. If you don't, you will fall back to the step you just left; that awful, uncertain *conscious ignorance*. What's the most important thing? That the wipes are easy to rinse? That the butt won't turn red? That we are caring for the environment? That it's practical for us? Or all of the above? Even though there isn't a huge problem, you should think it through. Take a stand. You might need to come up with arguments in order to explain and defend your choice.

You will soon return to conscious awareness, and eventually you will be at the top of the stairs on the *unconscious knowledge* step. You will change your baby's diaper, in the dark and half asleep, without even thinking of it. You just do it. At this stage, you aren't very dependent on what everyone else thinks because you found a way that works for you.

We don't want to make you anxious, but try to picture numerous knowledge stairs—one for each thing you are about to learn (sleeping very little at night, comforting, bathing, holding, refraining from satisfying your own needs first, feeding, etc.). Then take note of how you run, jump, fall, crawl up and down (mostly up) all those stairs. No wonder it's difficult being a parent sometimes! If it consoles you in any way, you can recognize that everyone around you is stumbling up and down in the same way. With this thought in the back of your mind, you can't deny that it feels great walking up the stairs. It's just as incredibly frustrating standing on the *conscious ignorance* step as it is wonderful to flourish on the *unconscious knowledge* step. This is when we have learned something new! Being on the bottom and top steps pretty much does the same thing for our conscious self, but the big difference is that we have grown a lot by the time we get to the top.

So, frustration can actually make us learn things and help us grow. Tell that to a sleep-deprived parent and you'll get punched. Frustration doesn't necessarily mean that you are in the middle of a learning process. You may currently be facing something that is overwhelming.

You might need support. You may need to compare yourself to other parents. Ask for help! Talk to wise people around you. Express what it is that you want! If you don't want advice, say so—otherwise, you are probably going to get it. The people around you want to help, but they may not realize what you need help with. And for all of those who love to throw around "good" advice: your intentions are certainly well-meant, but don't assume that others want it—give advice away like you would a gift, but ask the person if they want it first and don't be upset if the person declines. It's okay if I say that I just want you to listen to my whining for a while; or if I ask you to walk around with the stroller so that I can take a nap; or surprise me with something that will invigorate me; or tell me what you would have done if you were me; or give me three completely insane suggestions on what I could do. If you want a piece or two of advice—ask for it. You are free to ask whatever you want! You could get a no, but you've most likely made someone else happy by having given him or her the opportunity to help and grow. In addition, you have been brave and revealed your smallness.

By showing that you can be small as well as great, you can help other parents in their growing process. You're not alone in feeling that parenthood can be tricky at times. We initially wrote about how important it is for us as parents to actually help each other, and helping another parent can come in the form of you standing up for your own unusual methods. "At our place we wash the baby's bottom with a sheet of wet writing paper. We rip it up in order to remove the sharp edges. It works great! I've also heard that there are wipes made out of foam rubber, soft paper, and fabric, but it wasn't for us." Someone will be impressed, while another person will think you're crazy. So what? Think of how much fun we'll have when we start telling each other about the crazy things we do! Or when we start talking about our failures. "We tried wet writing paper when diapering. Eva brought the recycling box home from work, but it was a total fiasco. It worked great as a poo scraper, but you should have seen how difficult it was to flush it down the toilet." We will succeed sometimes and fail other times. We will have to deal with both setbacks and success. We can change our actions and ourselves in order to fit our aspirations. As much and as many times as we want! We need to celebrate and believe in ourselves, as well as celebrate and believe in others who do what they think is best, even when they fail. Doing this will definitely make us grow.

Doing something as a parent, traditional or contrary, will affect our children. When we decide to do things in a certain way as parents, we do it on various premises. It can revolve around us learning how to cope. Sometimes you need something to be useful, another time you need it to be simple, other times fun or cheap, but it always needs to be about making things as good as possible for our children. It usually turns out this way, but if it doesn't, we are quick to correct it, yet also quick to judge ourselves. Not being perfect in front of our kids can also be a good thing. What are we teaching our children when we stand up for what we believe in and the decisions we make? When we fail but are okay with our shortcomings and still love ourselves? When we find that other people's solutions seem exciting? When we are brave, leave our comfort zone, and maybe do something that we in our wildest imagination didn't think we would do? When we stand firm in the midst of everything else shifting when it would be easier to just go with the flow? When we go with the flow because we can't be bothered doing otherwise or don't think that it's important to resist? When we're doing our best? When we reveal our true colors?

That we are human beings!

What do you need to start doing in order to grow as a parent?

What do you need to stop doing in order to grow as a parent?

What do you need to do more of in order to grow as a parent?

What do you need to do less of in order to grow as a parent?

When do you do it?

CRAZY THOUGHT

I do what Pippi Longstocking did and it usually works out!

Sometimes I get sick of all the advice, opinions, and ideas from others. I might ask for someone's opinion and all of a sudden I am listening to half a novel's worth about how it should be done or the best way of doing it.

Kristina with Briana, age 2½.

I've always hated getting advice and suggestions without me asking for them. I have a really hard time listening to others' "best way," especially when they aren't interested in what I think, but they have their own agenda for providing the advice. They either think that they are great or they just want to hear their own voice and express their opinion.

I can figure things out myself and if I want help or advice, I'll ask for it. It's not that I think I'm a know-it-all and that I know how to do everything by myself, but let me make the decision. I am an adult.

Before I had children, I often chose not to listen when someone was giving me tips or advice; I just nodded a little and went merrily on my way. Very rarely did I have to resort to shouting when people didn't understand that they pushed my limit. I really don't want to be rude and I try to listen and engage and reject the advice if it isn't helping me. But I'd like to do it without stepping on anyone's toes.

Our pedantic neighbors often gave us advice and ideas after we had just moved in, but the advice was mostly about them wanting us to do things in a way that would satisfy their aesthetic needs.

Neighbor 1: "It would look great if the hedge was as tall as the mailbox." (Ours was about forty inches higher.)

"It sure would," I said with a smile and stayed in my deck chair. "But we have done well with the grass."

My philosophy has been to not dig too deeply into something, be friendly, and not to let the criticism and ideas of others faze me.

It worked well. Until I got pregnant. Suddenly we were hot prey for all those people who knew so much more than us. My own mother, my mother-in-law, our friends with and without kids—they all had opinions, suggestions, and advice that had to be heard. I'm wondering whether this was because I was a relatively young mother or if everyone else has had to deal with the same thing.

"Do not . . ."

"You must . . ."

"You should . . ."

"You also have to think about that . . ."

I felt quite vulnerable because here I was standing in the middle of something that was completely new to me, and everyone else knew so much more than me, and everyone also had their own opinions. There were always plenty of different answers to the same question, which resulted in even more questions, and both our heads were spinning around. What was the right answer, what was the wrong one?

We decided to use my old familiar trick, which is pretending to listen, but still doing what we think is best for us. It was our baby and our pregnancy, and we didn't want to ruin it by worrying and thinking about what we should do. Loads of women have been pregnant before me and so many children had been raised with or without outsider advice. It was us against the world.

We went to an ultrasound fairly late to make sure that the baby was developing as she should. Afterwards, we went out for food to celebrate that everything was looking great. As we were sitting down and looking at the menu, I noticed that the person sitting at the next table was being served a big piece of meat and I felt how my mouth was watering: I wanted meat!

"I want what he is having," I said, pointing at his plate.

The waiter took note and asked, "I assume you want it well-done?"

"No, medium," I said, looking quizzically at him.

"Well-done," said the waiter while glancing at my stomach.

"Medium," I repeated and glared at him.

I understand that he had good intentions and that pregnant women shouldn't eat raw meat, but I wanted a steak, not a shoe sole. That's why I ordered it.

My husband, Jacob, gave me the thumbs up—us against the world.

This is the way it has continued: everyone has an opinion, which is fine by me, but I decide that I will not worry unnecessarily.

I could make a long list of times I've used this strategy. During my pregnancy I met with three different midwives at the maternity clinic and they all said different things about weight and measurements and childbirth. I read up on it, asked the people I trusted, and tried what I felt was best, without worrying too much.

I was happy that we only had to meet with one midwife who gave us just the support we needed when giving birth. We had to manage by ourselves as far as we could take it, and then there she was by our side until it was over. What an experience.

Breastfeeding! How many different tips, tricks, advice, and recommendations are there?

I gave up on the whole demands-and-obligations list, and things just worked out by themselves. For me, it was about being able to relax, to forget about the methods and demands and to just be. It sounds like it was all sunshine, but naturally, even I worried about rashes, weight dips, and fevers, but I decided to always trust my own or Jacob's gut feeling, and tried not to listen too much to what others had to say. We are the ones who know best and most about our child.

We love her so much and we want the absolute best for her, so it can't really be frustrating.

It's us three against the world.

Then what happened?

Briana is now two and a half years old and in daycare, which is working great. She has been there for a year now and the staff is starting to understand us. In the beginning, there were a lot of implied comments about clothes and other things. All I want is clear communication where the staff tells me straight up what they do or don't want, not like at the start when they, with a smile and a tilted head, told me that Briana's pants were really nice, but perhaps not very practical, as they got dirty easily. As if I was less knowledgeable and didn't understand that dirt is more visible on light pants than on dark. It's my choice to do laundry; I want Briana to look nice and not have a problem with pants covered in sand and mud.

I prefer a clear: "We want to have Briana wear winter pants when it's muddy." I'll take that.

New thoughts

I never realized what a minefield having a child was—all the opinions and ideas coming at the prospective or new mother, even if you don't want them. You have to fit into this shared world: this is the way to do it, this is how you should be as a parent. It's not spoken of explicitly, but instead appears as advice or ideas, which elicits a sense of guilt when I don't do it right.

But what's the right thing to do?

I do what Pippi did and it usually works out!

There is no cheat sheet for parenting.

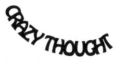

Giving Christmas away

The father of my children and I don't live together anymore, so we have split our furniture and other things and agreed on living arrangements during the weeks and weekends to make sure that we create the best situation for our children. But exactly how fair do we have to be?

Mia with Amanda, age 4, and Viktor, age 6.
For the first Christmas after our separation, we wanted to maintain the appearance that everything was okay and do things in the same manner as usual. It was sort of like we wanted to reassure ourselves, but also the children. *Everything is like it's always been, kids, the difference is that Dad and I are not living together anymore.* Ever since the children's father and I started dating, we have celebrated Christmas with his large family. His family is incredibly loving and kind and I've always felt welcome there. Christmas means everything to this loud family and everyone works hard at making sure traditions are kept alive. The Christmas tree is always in the same corner and the little Santa Claus stands behind the door and shows up at six o'clock on the dot, wearing the same suit as last year. This brings a sense of charm and assurance, even though it isn't necessarily my picture of a quiet and peaceful Christmas. Ever since my sister and I stepped into adulthood, my parents have spent all their Christmases abroad. We never made a big deal about Christmas in our family, not even when we were little. For that reason, we don't have many important Christmas traditions. So as the holidays approached after our separation, we went with our usual routine; we traveled there together, newly divorced, but on the surface we were

"fake friendly" to each other and happy with our "joint" decision about no longer living together. It certainly wasn't any fun for either one of us.

I felt that Mike's family was overly jaunty and sympathetic, acting like "it's so nice that we can all be friends after all." Everyone did their best to maintain the appearance of a Merry Christmas, but I just wanted to get out of there after the first day. I wanted to be back home, where I could stay inside and pull the covers over my head. The kids loved being there, they loved hanging out with all of their cousins, as well as their grandma and grandpa, so for them it was the best Christmas. They had everything they could ever want when it comes to a real family holiday, how could I take this tradition away from them? I was wrestling with myself during Christmas and I promised myself I would never go through with this experiment again.

The following year, we started planning for Christmas in October. I wasn't the one who brought it up. The children's father wondered whose turn it was to take care of the kids during Christmas, and if we should take turns every year like others do. Or if I, now that our separation had settled a bit, would go to his parents' home when it was my turn to take care of the kids. I was still very welcome and the whole family would really appreciate it if I came along.

I remember that I said I would think about it, because I really needed to figure out what I wanted to do. The previous Christmas was still a vivid reminder of what it was like forcing myself to be there. In a purely selfish manner, I really wanted to be only with my children on Christmas Eve. However, there is so much more to this holiday than this weekend. Christmas is so important to the children's father. For the kids, this is the only way to celebrate Christmas. It's a very special tradition that the grandparents create for their children and grandchildren. Could I really ruin it because of my egoistic thoughts?

The kids are very considerate when it comes to Mom and Dad, so they would surely understand. No one should be sad or alone. If Dad gets one Christmas, then Mom gets the next one, one for me and one for you, that's the way my children work anyway.

I called the children's father and gave him Christmas, which was completely crazy and unexpected. When I told him that I would get him a nice gift, I felt that I was doing the right thing. I gave it to him until further notice.

I told him why I made the decision and I hadn't heard him this happy in several years, not only happy but also incredibly grateful,

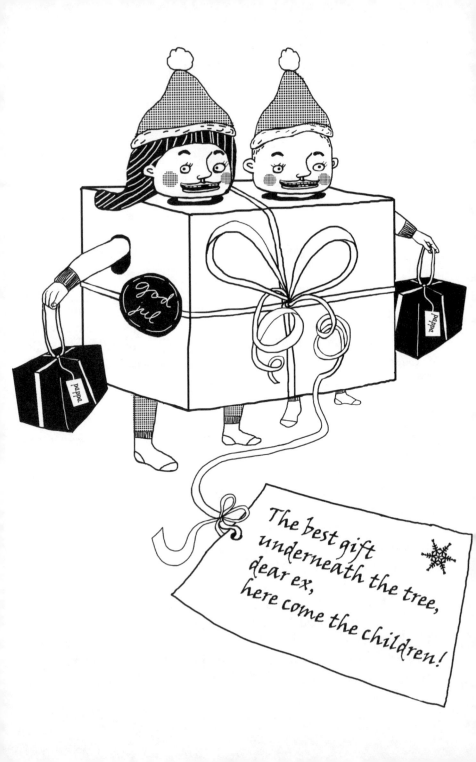

which I didn't really expect. I could also hear it in his voice that he felt sorry for me, but I could also sense that he respected me for my unselfishness. That was how I interpreted it anyway.

I told the kids that they would spend Christmas with their father and that it would be fun. That's when the questioning began, especially from Viktor: what I would do, why I didn't want to go, or if I wasn't allowed to go.

I told him that I could come along but that I didn't want to, because his father and I enjoy ourselves the most when we aren't around each other. I told him that I always think of them, that they will have a lot of fun with grandma and grandpa, and that I would spend time with my friend Nina because she was working in the barn during Christmas.

Then what happened?

This is our second year with this new tradition and I think it is working well. I can plan my Christmas according to when the kids are gone and they are now at peace with the fact that I celebrate Christmas elsewhere. The children's grandmother calls me every year and invites me, but I've kindly declined, which has probably been a relief for both of us. I don't want anyone to have a guilty conscience because of my decision, not my children nor their grandmother.

The kids and I have our own Christmas time, either before Christmas Eve or on New Year's Eve. We have our own traditions with tasty food and Christmas gifts. The reactions from others have been both positive and negative. A lot of people are very selfish when it comes to their children. But I want my children to grow and blossom, which means that I can't skimp on the sun and fertilizer.

New thoughts

Giving one Christmas away every other year has been a win-win for all of us. We are more generous to each other and the bitterness that I hear from other divorced parents doesn't exist between us. We don't work like that. However, I think there would have been a lot more competition about what's mine and what's his if I hadn't given Christmas away. Being generous makes me feel good and it will benefit my children.

CRAZY THOUGHT

I don't care about the baby!!!

When I came home from the maternity ward with baby number two, I felt a little concerned about what big brother would say about getting a sibling. But I couldn't have imagined how he would react. Before me would lie weeks of anger and resentment. My first-born began a boycotting campaign that makes me so sad. I try to coax, inveigle, and be a tactical parent, but what good does it do?

Åsa with Svante, 5 months, and Felix, age 3.

I think about parenting a lot: the way I would like to be, in what way I want to respond to my kids, and what's good for them. It may sound pretentious, but I'm interested in pedagogy as well as psychology, as I see them as two major ingredients in parenthood. It's not like I am constantly worrying any more than other parents would, but when we were expecting our second child, I had read a lot about what it might be like to have a new sibling.

With newfound knowledge, many sensible thoughts, and after a whole lot of discussions and researching with friends and acquaintances, I felt well prepared to become a mother of two. Felix was also as prepared as a three-year-old can be. We had read educational books on expecting and getting siblings to him—I don't really think that Felix understood most of it, because I barely did myself.

The delivery went well and it felt amazing when we found out it was a beautiful little boy—again. We talked with Felix on the phone and he sounded excited about getting a little brother. He was naturally curious and eager to greet his new brother whom we decided to name Svante. Björn, my husband, quickly went home to collect Felix, who had been with Grandma and Grandpa while we were in the hospital. I was a little nervous about Felix's arrival and prepared myself that it might be tough on him, and perhaps for me and Björn, as well. It had only been the three of us for three long, comfortable years. I had read somewhere that getting a sibling could be compared to me or Björn bringing home a new partner who would stay with us. I read it during an especially unstable period of my pregnancy and I remember that just the thought of Björn dragging home another girl made me bawl.

I had also read and heard that getting siblings usually works out just fine, and my common sense told me that everything would be okay considering how many non-disordered people with siblings there are on this earth. But I was prepared and Felix would be involved in changing diapers, having alone time with both Mom and Dad, and holding his little brother.

He was a little hesitant during that first meeting at the hospital, but both Björn and I felt that it went pretty well. And after a few pleasant days, it felt good to get back home. We didn't know what was lurking in the shadows.

After coming home, it all went downhill. Felix completely lost it and took it all out on me. He became extremely jealous, but he didn't take it out on Svante, he did the opposite. He was very nice and caring toward him and wanted to hold him in his arms, change his diapers, and sleep beside him. He didn't take it out much on Björn either. I, on the other hand, was cruelly set off to the side. Consistently and constantly. It was manifested in the form of: "Felix, Dad, and Svante—NOT Mom." "No, Mom don't sit here/come along/cook/eat/read the book/hug/swim/sing with us . . ." (pretty much all the activities that you can do together as a family). "Felix doesn't want Mom to change diapers/dress Svante/tuck him into bed . . ." "LEAVE, Mom!"

We tried everything that we had read or heard. We tried alone time with Felix and Mom, but he was either plain grumpy or he would scream for Daddy and Svante. We tried letting him decide—that is,

Mom agreed to be excluded and left to gripe in the kitchen. We had several nice "family talks" and so on.

But no, I wasn't worth anything in Felix's eyes.

One evening, when I once again tried to reclaim our nightly ritual of storytelling and singing, I was turned away with the words: "No, be with Svante instead. LEAVE!" and that was the end of all our rational attempts. I felt so sad and discouraged. It felt as if I (even though it had been the both of us) was the one who ruined everything by having Svante. I longed so much for Felix's love and what we had before Svante came along and ruined everything. As I was standing in Felix's doorway with tears in my eyes, Felix with a hostile look in his—eyes like laser beams—I gave up and burst out: "I don't care about this baby! I don't care about him! I want you, just you! Now!"

And in that moment everything changed—a miracle above all miracles—he looked at me with surprise, brought over his blanket, and lay down on my arm, content as before.

Then what happened?

After this outburst, Felix has not excluded me once. He may certainly be jealous of his little brother, but he expresses it in other ways. I feel personally that I have an easier time being myself around my children.

New thoughts

Being able to express what I really think and feel as a parent can do wonders. I am no more than who I am! Pedagogy and psychology are still interesting, but my common sense and my intuition are often more useful in practice. Also, I kind of think that Felix subconsciously forced me to react. It was like he was frustrated that Björn and I played the part of a happy family when we actually felt that it all was pretty radical, strange, and difficult.

Thank you for that lesson, Felix!

Pastries work wonders

The daycare our son attends had to relocate all of a sudden. Our son had made it very clear to us that he absolutely did not intend on attending the new kindergarten. We needed to work and had no choice but to send him to daycare. How would we be able to do this without forcing him?

Johan with Anton, age 3, Cal, age 7, and Billy, age 9.

I had been away for a while, and during that period, mold had been discovered in the building where Anton attended kindergarten. With just a few days' notice, we learned that the entire daycare would be relocated to another location a good distnace away from home. Anton is decisive and strong-willed and he told me straight away that he was not going to attend the new kindergarten.

I got back home that Sunday night and decided to be tactical; I would devote Monday to checking the new place out with Anton and to try to get him used to the thought of being there on the following Tuesday. It turned out that my tactics were useless, as Anton still refused to go to kindergarten. Okay, I thought, and forged on. I will have to use other methods. Bribes! Said and done. I proposed a new, genius idea to Anton: *This is probably the best daycare because on the way to it, there is a bakery where a baker works and he makes pastries and cookies.* We could stop by every morning and try a new kind of pastry.

I was a bit worried that I had painted myself into a corner and would now be forced to buy pastries every morning for an eternity. But I didn't really have the time to be concerned about this at that point; I just needed a quick solution.

Anton was excited by the proposal and the next day we began to try the entire assortment, starting off with a cinnamon bun. We passed the bakery every morning and Anton tried the vanilla wafers, danishes, doughnuts, cookies, and tarts. The tarts were the best.

Even though we found a great solution that really worked, I was fighting feelings of guilt that it was not healthy to eat sweets each day. On the other hand, I don't think it made a big difference if my children wanted to eat buns every morning. I could see how it solved our problems for the time being and I knew the kids were getting what they needed. Still, I felt compelled to explain myself to the bakers and tell them that Anton had a hearty breakfast in the morning and that this was only temporary. I wonder how much they really cared?

Once I told the team of bakers that I met hordes of perfect parents on their way to kindergarten with their perfect children. I could almost read the speech bubbles above their heads: "A bun every morning! Probably because the dad is stressed and doesn't think to feed the kid a proper breakfast! The sugar will corrode his teeth!" I wanted a jacket with a sign on the back that read: "I have given my children a proper breakfast, time, love, I have brushed their teeth, given them neat and clean clothes . . . and we're actually just doing this for a short period of time to overcome the obstacle of Anton not wanting to attend his new kindergarten . . . that he had to move to because the old one was moldy . . . and it's nothing that we can control."

Ridiculous! I thought I was being incredibly slick and quick-witted when I came up with the perfect solution. Yet, on our way to the kindergarten, I had to slow down, making sure that the bun was eaten before we arrived and all the perfect parents and perfect staff wouldn't catch on to what was happening. And I carefully wiped the crumbs around Anton's mouth.

I can say with certainty that pastries really did work wonders, since Anton agreed to go to his new kindergarten without feeling sad.

Then what happened?

Anton got sick of eating buns and tarts every morning. We discovered a new route where there was ice "growing" on the hill, which he found much more exciting. Nowadays, he attends daycare as usual, sometimes with more eagerness, and other times with less.

New thoughts

Bribes work! Although I've known that for a while. Bribing your children is considered to be a cheap trick, but why make it harder than it needs to be? I am a resourceful parent who helps my children. Other parents think that it was a fun and clever idea. Maybe I have helped someone else to do the contrary. Next time I will do it with my head up high and without brushing away the crumbs around Anton's mouth.

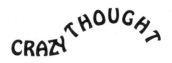

To choose one child

I don't like being pregnant. I have problems falling asleep at night and I don't like going on maternity leave. One child is perfect for us, but our friends and family seem to think otherwise. I feel stressed and pressured when I think about the fact that we probably should have more children.

Linda with Agnes, age 4.

Kent and I had had been living together for a year when we started talking about having children. Or more so, that we couldn't picture ourselves growing old without children. So really, there was no strong desire right there and then. Life was fairly routine and our egos were becoming too big. We simply wanted to grow something other than ourselves.

When I was expecting with Agnes, I remember that we discussed the fact that we knew nothing about having children. We didn't really plan much at all. We were about to have one child and the *idea* of having more children in the future didn't exist. It was just the idea of having more children. Agnes was born and we quickly became aware of what it meant to be a parent. We obviously loved Agnes and were happy to have her, but we also thought it was pretty tough. For me, being up at night was a practical problem. I don't do well on too little sleep and I really suffered from a lack of it. I took the first half of my maternity leave and I thought it was really boring. I'm used to variation, tempo, and intellectual challenges. That's sort of everything a maternity leave isn't, for me anyway.

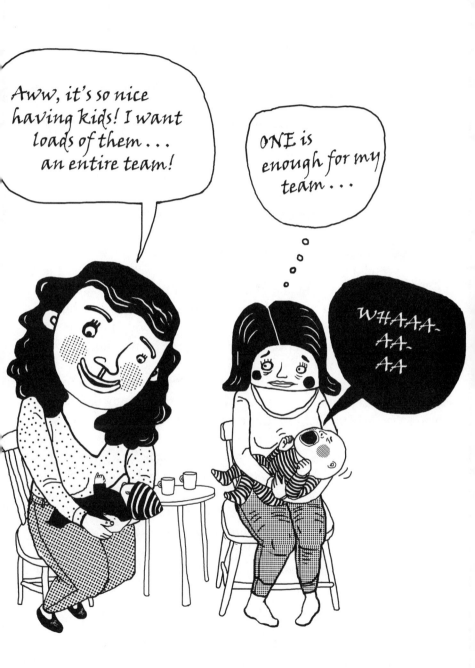

We started talking about only wanting to have one child after our parental leave. We didn't really make any decisions, but agreed that we would have more children if we wanted to (which sounds pretty obvious). I subsequently didn't feel like having more children and I wrestled a lot with questions about why I felt this way. I wanted to have the will! People around us started asking if we were going to have more kids, but I'd be lying if I said that someone specifically pressured us. I felt pressure, but I'm not sure where it came from.

I have read and heard about the benefits of having siblings. What would happen to Agnes if we didn't give her any brothers or sisters? Would she become a social freak? I saw before me a lonely Agnes, with no other relatives other than her own parents. So lonely and sad in a way . . . and it was so incredibly selfish of us to opt out of giving her a sibling just because we didn't want more children.

I was thinking and thinking, and no matter which way I sliced it, I still didn't want more children. Luckily, Kent and I felt the same way. It made us strong in our belief that we wouldn't have any more children, other than if we wanted to—selfish or not, what does it matter? Egotistic or not, what makes people choose to have more children? When I posed this question to my friends who had more than one child, they gave me responses like "I had more love to give," or "we wanted our children to have siblings." The answers made my already bad feelings worse. No one said that they chose to have children for their own sake.

I still wonder why it's so common to have two children. If you look around, you'll discover that a lot of things are made for a family of two adults and two children. If you try to find a trip and accommodations, it becomes very clear, as there are often family packages meant for four people. Before the seven-seater cars, the maximum number of children that could fit in the car was three. Say what you want, but I think people are more pragmatic than they realize, and the number of children you choose to have is to some extent controlled by what's practical.

Then what happened?

Agnes has grown older and being a parent is starting to feel more and more comfortable. Now we can do more things together that amuse me as an adult. We can hold a conversation that I can gain something from. My contemplations have given me a sense of calm. I feel good about having one child. It suits our family and our mentality. We like small groups where we get the time to talk and have time for ourselves. We have realized that we aren't "the-more-the-merrier" family. We can only handle a small number of people.

A friend of mine, who also thinks the early childhood years are difficult, is expecting her second child and said, "Now we will have a couple of stressful years." Some people think that it sounds crazy, but I respect her and her husband's choice and approach to parenting. They want more children but find young children difficult. They do somehow see that it's all worth it, though. Honestly and consciously. Yes, perhaps I could have another child, if it was possible to get a three-year-old right off the bat. I don't want anymore of the tough years!

New thoughts

We have chosen one child because it suits us. The road to that realization has been long. It feels real. In the same way that I've been looking, listening, and speaking things that confirmed my fears about the "lonely" child, I can choose to find things that confirm my positive thoughts. It's easy to get stuck in thinking that I have to conform to norms, but that can be just as bad. As a parent, I have the right to make my own choices!

From burned out to fired up

I've gone from being a creative and independent human being to a completely self-effacing parent. I have been completely burned out by my parental chores. I almost hate my family and I'm going to diiieee soon!

Helen with Matilda, age 2, and Viktor, age 6.

The new year began in the worst possible way. Matilda got chickenpox and horrible, festering sores all over her body. She cried and tore the skin off and couldn't understand why her parents nagged her about the scratching. The medicine helped somewhat, but at times she was drowsy and needed a lot of nurturing. I was planning on working during the holidays, but that turned into taking care of my of sick child instead. *Oh well,* it probably didn't really matter. I figured that the office was still quite empty with everyone taking off, and that we could probably ride out the chickenpox. My heart ached from seeing our daughter feeling so awful and not being able to provide more comfort and help other than hugs and love.

Matilda was sick for over two weeks. Her recovery took longer than we expected, and it took even longer for the infection to completely disappear. Mike had many meetings and I actually earned less money than he did, so me being home seemed like the sensible decision. I often worked from home, so I was able to use some sick days interspersed with working from home. I think Mike was at home for two whole days during Matilda's illness. That was fine with me.

She attended kindergarten for two days when Viktor came down with the chickenpox next. I almost started to cry when I saw the all-too-familiar rash that suddenly appeared everywhere on his body. A slightly selfish thought popped into my head—couldn't they have gotten the chickenpox at the same time at least? But I quickly pushed that thought away. The situation was what it was and I simply had to be patient.

Strangely enough, I offered to stay home again. I've always been more distressed than Mike and I thought if I was home, I would at least be able to check up on Viktor instead of sitting at work and worrying. Silly, I know! And a really poor argument in the long run, because the course of this chickenpox was as bad as the last one. It actually almost felt worse having the older child suffering from it since he could actually express how he felt about the pain and itchiness. I couldn't get a good night's sleep and I barely left the house. Normally I would always feel the need to get away, take a walk, or go to the gym, but I did nothing. When Viktor slept or watched a movie, I sat at the computer and worked. My whole existence revolved around the guilt I felt of not doing enough. I felt exhausted and didn't have enough energy to get in touch with friends and family. The tiredness made me irritable and I would snap at the children. At the same time, I felt ashamed of myself. I wasn't fed up with the kids; it was the whole awful situation that made me so tired.

One may ask where Mike was during the duration of this. Was he an absent jerk of a husband? Not at all, he was concerned and felt bad about the children's illnesses as much as I did. The difference was that he had a social life. And he could easily put aside his concerns when he was away from home. He has always had the easy attitude that you gain nothing from being stressed. But I couldn't relate to that frame of mind.

When Viktor started to recover, Matilda got an ear infection. She cried and was in terrible pain, and even though I almost broke inside, I had to appear to be energetic and strong for the kids. Our neighbor took care of Viktor while I took Matilda to the emergency room. The kids and I were actually home alone, as Mike was in England for a one-week course. A course that I nearly forced him to attend—it was an opportunity that he couldn't miss out on. I wanted to prove that I could do it all on my own. Because . . . well, I don't really know why. I thought I was a rational and intelligent person. Or was I? From somewhere inside, a Stone Age monkey brain whispered to me that sick children need their mother at all costs. But it was actually me who needed them, and during this period I had developed some sort of need for martyrdom for an unknown reason. Did I think that someone would see my sacrifices, pat me on the back, and say "good girl"?

Matilda quickly felt better after she started taking penicillin. I was the one who was completely falling apart. Mike phoned from England and asked if he should come home, but I said that everything was under control. I lied.

When my husband finally arrived on Sunday evening, I broke down completely. I remember I had to hold onto the sink so that I wouldn't collapse from the crying, and I could barely answer his question as to what was wrong. The only thing I could utter was that I couldn't do it anymore.

My astute family tucked me in on the couch and Mike told the kids that I was tired and needed rest. Then he called my mom and asked her if she would be willing to go on a one-week trip with me. Maybe borrow her colleague's summerhouse in Denmark? I heard him say that it was an absolute emergency.

And it was. Had I stayed home another day, I don't know what I would have done. I was sick and tired of illnesses, family, and myself, and I longed for somewhere else. How we, how I, ended up here, I really didn't know. We just got stuck in a rut because it was comfortable, I guess. Why didn't I fight for my right to a social life outside of my home? For my right to go to work? I probably wouldn't have had to fight, I would have simply had to ask for it.

Instead, I got a wonderful week in a beautiful house on the west coast of Jutland. With a supportive mother, who had the decency to be silent when I needed it, and let me talk when I wanted to. Life was amazing, even though it was windy and low season, just because it was something different than home. We walked and talked and cooked and laughed. I was slowly healing. And I didn't miss my family once.

Then what happened?

When I got home, we naturally hugged and hugged for a while. I had gotten just enough of my very own time to feel like a person again. I realized that this chain of events was largely the result of an unfortunate coincidence, but it was also due to my own behavior. The children have remained relatively healthy for several years since. And if they have ever had to stay home from daycare or school, Mike and I have shared the responsibility of staying home with the sick kids. Strictly and with precise justice.

I'm someone who needs a lot of time outside the house, which seems to bother some people. A colleague of mine (who also has children) told me yesterday that she thinks that I'm constantly participating in outside activities. The accusatory tone in her voice was perhaps only envy. I actually don't care what she or others think—there is no one who knows the history of my family and what we have gone through. I stand for what I do, and yes, I regularly go to the cinema or a restaurant with my friends. Because I want it and I need it.

But in between, I am at home and I'm an awesome mom with the strength to love my family.

New thoughts

Having my own space is vital for me. Caring for sick children for six weeks in almost total isolation is a real health hazard. I will never let something like that happen again. My family feels the same. I need to take great responsibility for myself in order to feel good. There lives an "I can do it myself" attitude in me and it has gained quite a lot of weight. Sometimes it gets in the way when I need to ask for help. We are becoming friends again though—I am the one who decides!

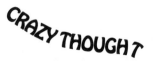

Running away from the family

How can one believe that three adult siblings with their parents and separate families could be able to share a medium-sized cottage without harming each of the relationships? It personally drives me crazy.

Maria with Teo, age 3½, Marianna, age 5, and Tad, age 7.

I am married and, therefore, don't have much say when it comes to my husband's inseparable family—that's how I feel anyway. As long as we have been together, my in-laws and Cal's siblings expect us to stay at the cottage for at least two weeks every summer. It was pretty relaxing before we had children, as they didn't expect much from me. I could lie down and read a book or go somewhere else if it got too noisy. But after we had three children in rapid succession, I have spent more time babysitting, time managing, and house-sitting during those two weeks. The fact is that this cottage is a ton of work. It's like a two-week labor camp: if you aren't felling trees, you are painting the fence or something needs to be sealed, repaired, or fixed. My two sisters-in-law and I baby-sit and assist in the kitchen, and our husbands labor with their father and fathers-in-law. Their mother is in the kitchen ensuring that meals and snacks are served at the right times and she compiles a long to-do list for these two weeks of summer.

This is their idea of the perfect way to spend time together; it's important to work together and it's crucial to have the right roles. The children enjoy seeing their cousins and I get on well with the whole family, but after about a week, I start feeling very irritated. The children's grandparents own the house, but it's implied that we're doing all of this grunt work for the future, when the three siblings will own the place. The property and labor is equally shared.

Cal isn't interested in sharing this place with his siblings, but the work that he is doing is for his parents. We've talked a lot about this and agreed that the healthy relationship that we have with his siblings and their families wouldn't benefit from a common ownership. We've only had three weeks of vacation all together over the last two summers. In order to coordinate our everyday lives with a kindergarten that's closed for summer, we have tried a lot of different options and nearly drove ourselves mad just spending two-thirds of the duration of our time together with a whole bunch of other people, when what we really needed is our own family time.

Last summer was the last straw, as we had a tough spring with a lot of the children being sick, parental leave, and demanding work schedules. Cal almost lost it from exhaustion and too much work, so with my cheerful support, he phoned his parents and stated very clearly that we needed a real vacation if we were to come out to the countryside. That we would come to spend time with family, help out with small things, and so that the children could see their cousins and grandparents. I was very straightforward, very clear. It felt good. When we arrived at the house and parked the car, we noticed a pile of building materials. The house would be getting a new roof and my husband would build it with the help of his brother and brother-in-law. I felt sad and dejected, and Cal was furious. It was the first time I had seen him that angry with his parents, and he yelled and complained and finally we got into the car and left. It was like a scene out of a family drama: grandmother crying, children crying, me being speechless and just looking straight ahead while Cal muttered aloud to himself. We sped off in our car and were gone.

But where were we going? We didn't want to go back to the cottage and the chores again, nor did we want to go back to our home in the stuffy city; so we suddenly found ourselves on a road trip through the country with three small children. It lasted five days; we lived in motels and rooms for rent. We visited friends whom we hadn't seen in several years. We had lots of fun and were on an adventure with our children. We didn't talk to Cal's parents during those five days; we didn't call and neither did they. But we still wanted to be with our family and the children longed for all their cousins, so we decided to go back on the last day and mend fences with everyone. It was now or never.

Cal talked to his siblings and parents and told them how he felt and he expressed his thoughts on working on the house. He also raised the issues of what a burden it was for everyone if all they did was work, and he pointed out that summer and spending time with the kids was more important to us than the old house.

Then what happened?

We will spend one week in the house with cousins and grandparents this summer. Then we are going to travel by car and stay at a motel with the kids; we are all really looking forward to it. They have talked a lot about our road trip last summer; it was really an adventure for them to see new places, and we knew we had to do that again. There might be work to be done, as grandfather has asked what Cal is willing to help out with, and there is a lot of work that goes into an old house. But he will ask, and I think Cal will speak up, if the only thing he is needed for is work. I hope he does.

New thoughts

It's so hard saying no to someone, especially to those who are closest to us. It's also hard to be receptive to others' needs, even if they are clearly stated.

Our road trip was the beginning of something better for us as a family, as we got to experience new things together. It also affected the communication between Cal and his parents, because they realized how he really felt.

Gummy bears save dinner

I'm usually very paranoid that my kid will have a fit at the grocery store. I have seen other children lie on the floor plenty of times and just scream because they didn't get candy or something else they wanted. My fear is that I'm the one standing there, and it's my crazy child lying on the floor.

Anders with Lina, age 3.

I don't really know why I'm so nervous about bringing children with me when going shopping. The reason may be that before I had Lina, kids who screamed in the store really annoyed me. I remember thinking that there must be something wrong, either with the kids or with the parents. How hard could it be? I had many opinions in general on how parents should handle their children, and that's probably why it makes me so nervous now, as I have become a father myself. I've been so critical, which means that I have to live up to my own ideals, right?

At the same time, maybe I can be forgiven now? I have stopped with my negative thinking about other parents and I understand that they are doing the best they can. I also do the best I can and it's only right that I treat myself fairly.

Normally we go grocery shopping almost every day on the way home from daycare. I'm aware that it might not be the best idea. It's surely better to buy in bulk once a week and maybe leave Lina at home with one of us. We just don't ever get around to it, though. We live in the center of town where there are few supermarkets with not a lot of deals

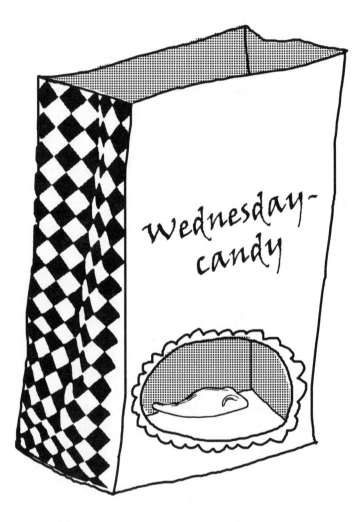

for buying in bulk, and that is the point of doing it, to save money. We don't have a car either and it would be hell carrying home bags and getting our arms stretched out at least four inches. Another problem is the fact that our fridge is suitable for a bachelor. Need I explain further why we don't buy in bulk? I can continue to carry on in this manner, apologize, and explain the choices I make as a parent, although in theory I think I have made amends for my previous parental disregard.

Yes, we presently shop every day on the way home from daycare, which puts us at higher risk for a mishap, because both Lina and I are very tired and hungry. We've never actually had a mishap at the store, but it's bound to happen! When Lina was two-and-a-half years old, I decided then to be mentally prepared when the time came. If things got bad, I would quickly offer her candy. I felt so much calmer, just having a plan. Nothing could stop us now. I was the king and Lina was my princess and we would be able to bring home food to the queen of the castle, effortlessly. It didn't matter that I paid the price with gummy bears.

I told my wife about my idea and she thought it was great. That made it seem even better and I decided to actually bring the matter up the next time Lina and I went shopping. Just as we were about to reach the checkout line and were standing in front of the candy section, I said, "We are getting some candy, too. One gummy bear for you, one for Dad, and one for Mom." Lina had tasted candy before, since we hang out with her older cousins a lot so she knew what it was and lit up. The checkout process was a breeze and on the way home she sat in her stroller and sucked on her precious, tasty, and colorful gummy bear. As soon as we got home, Mom received her gummy bear along with an account of our adventure.

Then what happened?

Lina is three years old now and we have continued giving her the gummy bears. Only positive things have arisen from it. For starters, our daily routine is smoother. Secondly, Lina is moderately interested in sweets at other times. When she attends a party and gets a bag of candy, she usually takes one piece, usually the gummy bear, eats it, and then she puts the bag aside.

I also think it's clever that we always just buy three pieces, one for each of us, as it isn't possible to get more—that's all there is in the bag. Lina has now started to choose her gummy bear herself. It's not so much about the fact that it's candy I think, as it is the nice colors. Some days she takes ages in deciding which color she wants.

Although I am pleased with our solution, I would still like to tell you that we eat very nutritious food and we brush our teeth, morning and evening. But, as I said, this is mostly stemming from my anxiety. Most people we've talked to think that it's a clever idea. Others have been skeptical and told me that they are dead set against giving their children candy. Sure, if it works for them, that's great—I think to myself, non-judgmental man that I am.

New thoughts

Gummy bears work well in our family. I am proud to have come across such a clever idea. I have a new theory that helps me in many situations: things that are prohibited often create fixations. If you allow things in small doses, it doesn't become such a big deal. It's like a vaccine. I have a friend who wasn't allowed to watch TV when he was a kid and you know what? He works in television today. Get it? My theory is legit.

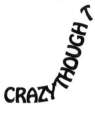
CRAZY THOUGHT

Climate smart

We live in a part of the country where it's pretty much unbearable to be outside during the winter. I've really tried to make the best of it, but it doesn't work—I hate being outside during winter! There is one simple reason—it's miserable! It's cold, dark, wet, and extremely depressing. Children and bad weather don't go together either, and during winter I'm faced with hell every morning. Science has made it possible for us to travel to the moon and transplant hearts, but time has been standing still when it comes to rain coats. They are just as ridiculously useless as they were when I was little.

In short: All outdoor activity between November and February—make that March—is totally overrated in my opinion!

Caroline with Agnes, age 3, Karin, age 5, Eleanor, age 10, and Pete, age 13. If I was living alone, I think I would stay inside the house all winter. Most things can actually be done by computer or phone. I remember in seventh grade my friend and I decided we would stay home from school whenever it was raining outside. People didn't understand us since it rained quite often, but now I'm an adult and I can decide for myself. . . . It would be against the norm to take a time-out from work and school and just stay inside during the cold months, so we decided to try staying inside on evenings and weekends. If it proved successful, we could step it up next winter.

When November rolled around, we hunkered down in our house; we lit candles, watched movies, and snuggled on the couch. We also spent time playing board games, video games, reading books, taking baths, having long conversations with each other, snacking, and cooking delicious meals together. It was really nice, but our younger children would sometimes ask us if they could go outside. They were obviously allowed and because our yard is fenced off, they could go outside and enjoy it by themselves (on the condition that they put on their outdoor clothing without our help). The older kids were delighted that they didn't have to leave the house. My husband and I could finally relax on the weekends.

The horrible process of dressing the kids on weekday mornings was still the same: fleece, jumpsuits, raincoats, hats, and waterproof gloves. I really came close to having a nervous breakdown after going through that each day. Our five-year-old would throw a fit every time she had to put on her rain gear, and our three-year-old cried "stop it, stop it" while my husband and I held her firmly to make sure that she got all her clothes on. I would switch from being infuriated to being in tears in seconds. When we finally managed to dress them and leave the house, it would be pouring outside! The three-year-old didn't seem to mind, despite the fact that she was in hysterics earlier—how does that work? The three-year-old is something of an outdoorsman, and likes, even loves, the fresh air; but the five-year-old starts feeling depressed, hates the heavy winter clothing, and has a very low SOC (sense of coherence). When we arrived at kindergarten and she found out that they were going to be playing outdoors (what a surprise—since they're outside every day . . .) she exclaimed, "Mom, I actually think it's crazy to be outside when it's raining!"

Then what happened?

We still don't like being outdoors during the winter season. I've also discovered that we don't like going outside during the summer if rain gear is necessary. What if it simply all comes down to the clothes? I find it hard to picture me changing my opinion on global warming. I was truly born in the wrong type of climate. I can picture us spending winters in a warmer place, after the children grow up and move out. It's such a discomfort staying inside for such a long part of the year.

New thoughts

Spending time inside on rainy days works great and we will continue doing that. There should be a kindergarten that's specialized in indoor activities: "The Daycare of Cuddling Indoors," "The Warm & Dry Daycare," "Indoor Joy Daycare," "The Anti-Raincoat Daycare." That lack of anxiety that comes with staying indoors far outweighs the unfulfilled need for daylight and fresh air.

I am also pleased that I have taken a stand on the issue of climate change. As a result, I don't have to complain about it as much as I used to. Then there's the issue of getting enough sunlight, which is probably pretty important, but I've read that it can be solved with special lights . . . if it weren't for the kids.

The luxurious lunch

Being on parental leave with a baby can be wonderful . . . but it can also be very tedious, boring, and lonely. Everything revolves around my child's various needs. What happens to my needs?

Jaclyn with Elsa, age 3.
When Elsa was a baby, I was the one who went on parental leave. Thomas, Elsa's father, worked and had to travel a lot, and he wasn't particularly engaged in our family life. This resulted in me having to deal with the responsibility of taking care of Elsa on my own for long periods of time. At first, I felt so fulfilled by being a mother, and even though it was hard, it was wonderful for the most part. But as time passed, I started feeling incredibly lonely. Everything I did, I did it with Elsa, and for the most part, I didn't interact with any other adults.

Fortunately, this changed when I started attending meetings for mothers at the Child Health Center. I met other moms there and we quickly formed a group of three who met almost every day. I soon realized that they were feeling lonely too, but there was one major difference: they had husbands who came home to them at night, while I usually spent my evenings alone with Elsa. We talked a lot about the importance of taking a break during the day. For a parent with a young child, every day can seem routine and the days all blend together, but at the same time, it's difficult to get together with other adults. We found that we really did need to put a cherry on top of our day, and socializing with adults was the perfect reward.

Because our group of mothers spent a lot of time together, we ended up having the same routines and our children started developing similar personalities. It started as early as when our babies were about six months old and we got them to sleep in the middle of the day. This meant that we had two hours to ourselves when we could "forget" that we were parents and we could just be ourselves. We then started to plan for luxurious lunches with wine for when we stopped breastfeeding. So about a month later, we put our fantastic idea into motion, which would give us something special to look forward to. We took turns arranging the lunches. We met every Wednesday at each other's homes on a rotating schedule. Whoever was the hostess for the week made the food and provided the wine. The guests brought their babies and showed up to an already set table. We started by putting the kids to bed and when they were asleep, it was our turn to have fun. It was so incredibly pleasant to sit down with two of my best friends, with good food and a bottle of wine. We really enjoyed those two hours, and when the kids woke up, we were like new mothers. We felt such an incredible sense of freedom and the wine made us feel a little more relaxed, too. It was the closest thing to luxury that existed in my life at that point, and boy, did I need it!

Our lunches led to various reactions from other mothers, and many reacted negatively to the fact that we drank wine. *My God*, we drank one bottle between us! It wasn't like we were getting drunk. One mother asked me indignantly, "Who takes care of the kids while you're doing your stuff?" Doing what stuff? Having a fun and pleasant time, or what? Since when had that become sinful?

Thomas also asked me at some point if it really was "appropriate" to drink wine with your friends when you're on maternity leave. Well, if you put it that way, I don't really feel that good about it. But I've never actually felt guilty because of it. My everyday life was boring and it meant a lot to me to spend time with my girlfriends, and the nice food and wine made it even better. You just can't have a bad conscience about that!

Then what happened?

Thomas is home a lot more these days and we often spend time with my lunch buddies and their respective families. We have a lot of fun together. The kids know each other and are becoming very close. We have gone from lunches to dinners, and we always take turns, so we're regularly in each other's homes. We still enjoy nice food accompanied by good wine. The children fall asleep together and they seem happy with that. Elsa sometimes gets mad when we wake her up and take her home in the stroller. It's the fifteen minutes of screaming that sometimes makes me wonder if it's okay to wake a child in the middle of the night, just because we adults enjoy spending time together. It feels odd putting your own adult needs ahead of your child's needs, but Elsa still enjoys it and doesn't seem too bothered by it.

New thoughts

My needs are important too! And what does my child really need? I assume that she has certain needs that aren't as big of a deal as I thought they were. A happy parent is a good parent. I am the best mother for Elsa.

Too tired to give yet another pat on the back

My husband and I feel physically and mentally exhausted, and after giving all of our energy to the kids, we have already used up all of our devotion and tenderness. Displaying affection and desire for one another feels like an obligation. Does that mean that our love is gone?

Jenny with Anthony, age 4, Erika, age 6, and Emily, age 7.

For a period of time when the children were younger, it literally felt as if they were sucking our blood. Both Robert and I were really tired since the kids needed our attention during every waking moment, and even when we were sleeping.

Raising three children who were so close in age was a task with consequences that we initially weren't aware of—for starters, all the logistical work surrounding food, talk, breastfeeding, diapers, clothing, laundry, strollers, kindergarten, getting in and out of the car, and on top of that, all the time that's needed for comforting, cuddling, patting, caring, and tolerating. Their need for love and intimacy was endless and never ceased; they were by our side day and night. The three of them slept together in our bed for long periods of time, so there we were; like one big family of pigs, trying to sleep. I would often wake up in some part of the house, not knowing where I was, but there was always a child who had followed me during my sleep walking, lying next to me. I was sick of my children, I couldn't even look at my husband, and I wished for a little cabin in the woods where I could just be by myself.

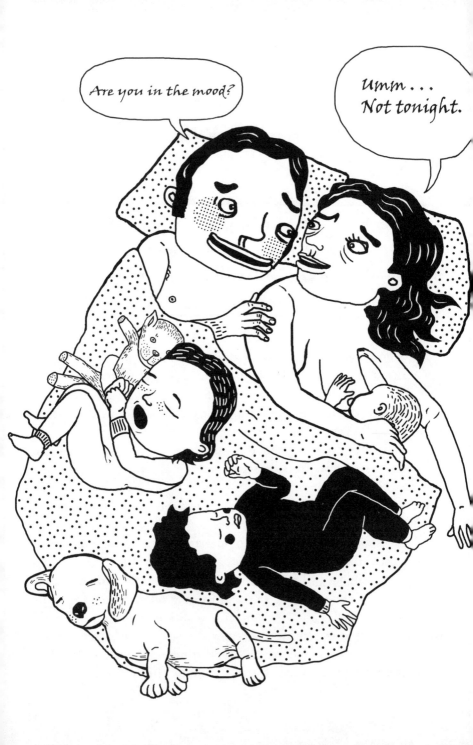

The sad part was that we, Robert and I, had stopped talking to each other. We had always talked about everything, but we didn't even have the energy to do that anymore. The physical bit was the same; our sex life was non-existent and even intimacy was just out of the question.

Mostly, I felt that there was a sense of if you pat me, I'll pat you back. Robert felt the same way; one of us would occasionally be in the mood, but we never coordinated with each other. After I tried to seduce him a few times and he responded with an indifferent yawn, or he came up with the boring suggestion spending a little "time" together (which I normally wouldn't mind), our love life was pretty much non-existent. Or, more precisely, it was stone dead.

I was starting to have fears: we should be having a sex life, we should hunger for each other and at least meet each other's needs for closeness and tenderness, because if that isn't alive, our relationship is dead.

I remember sitting at a friend's house, reading a sex column in some crappy magazine. It dealt with parents finding time for sex during the toddler years and I remember how upset the suggestions made me. The article stated that caressing and giving each other tenderness and love would bring about an active sex life.

But for us, it didn't matter whether I touched his knee or a more intimate spot, the issue was the lack of closeness and tenderness.

I could barely keep up with my own needs and fulfill my own desires, so how was I supposed to fulfill someone else's needs?

I was beyond satisfied with the tenderness and intimacy from my three amazing parasites who nearly lived inside my skin.

One day, we went to the zoo and I still carry the memory of something that happened that day.

The children's favorite part of the trip was when they got to play with some of the farm animals; they ran after goats, sheep, and pigs and cuddled and petted them. In the corner lay a giant sow with at least eight piglets jumping all around her and I felt so bad for her. When would she be able to breathe?

On the wall above there was a notice with instructions not to pet the sow. I read it out loud to Emily and Erika who followed up with the obvious "Why?"

While I was explaining it to them, I realized that I was talking about myself. The mother pig needs to be by herself. She provides so much food and love that she's too exhausted to be petted anymore. She needs to spend time alone, to have the strength to spend time with all of her kids.

"So when the piglets grow up and learn how to eat by themselves, she'll want to be petted again?" asked Emily.

"Sure," I said.

We were staying at a hotel and while our whole herd of piglets was sleeping in the other room, I relayed to Robert my conversation with Emily and told him that I sort of felt like the sow lying in the corner. Then Robert made a joke about him being the boar who was also tired of the piglets and he just wanted his wonderful life of playing in a puddle of mud back. And for the first time in a very long time, we were joking with each other, talking about ourselves rather than the kids, and I really felt that we were back to being ourselves again.

Robert summed up our relationship perfectly. He felt that we should be comfortable in the fact that we actually loved each other and wanted to live together, and we really had a strong connection, it was just that there was a recession going on at the moment.

Our physical needs existed, but right now they were tucked in and sleeping, which was good since they got to rest, and they would awaken later and not be tired.

I liked that idea.

We also decided to have a month of letting each other be, which meant that neither one of us would in any way try to get the other's attention when it came to cuddling, snuggling, back scratching, kissing, or sex. If we wanted something, we had to deal with it ourselves.

We realized this was harder than we thought when we noticed that all along we were actually trying to get each other's attention by putting a hand on the other's back, brushing each other's cheeks, or holding hands when we ended up at the bottom of our piglet pile.

Then what happened?

Our "leave each other alone" month ended up stretching for a couple more. We talked a lot about what we needed and didn't need. We didn't actually forbid anything, but it was nice living together without any pressure and demands. We have always been very physical with each other and we need physical contact in order to feel good, but it was such a relief not to feel obligated and able to say that I didn't want to hold his hand, because I would die if another person touched me at that moment.

He didn't feel rejected because he knew that this was about me and my need for solitude, not me thinking he was a disgusting, hairy boar.

New thoughts

I've thought a lot about love, intimacy, and sexuality. To me, intimacy and sexuality are about satisfying my own primary needs, sleeping well, spending time on my own, and ensuring that my body and soul aren't exhausted. If all of this is intact, I blossom and I have so much to give to others. But at the same time, there are so many musts that I still read about in magazines:

Find intimacy with your partner!

Have a good sex life after having kids!

Find the spark in your relationship!

These kinds of headlines only make me feel uneasy and probably instill a bad conscience in many others who don't really feel up for it.

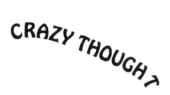
Outsource your walk with the stroller

As a parent, I feel frustrated that I always have to do everything myself and I never have time to even open a newspaper, go to the bathroom, or finish a thought. It feels like I've lost myself between the couch and changing table and I have an ongoing inner monologue nagging me about the injustices, inequality, and imbalance in my life.

All I want to do is hide under a blanket and not go out for walks with my baby because I don't even have enough energy to push the stroller to the elevator. Meanwhile, my bad conscience appears like a letter in the mailbox: Fresh air is good for children! Children need fresh air!

What do you do when reality and the romanticized notions of being a parent don't match?

Lena with Oleg, age 2½.
During Oleg's first six months, I was so tired at times, that after feeding and diapering him in the middle of the night, I couldn't fall back asleep like he did. What a pain it was to lie on the bed waiting, wide-awake, for

the next breastfeeding time. I twisted and turned; sounds that came from my husband and son annoyed me, I couldn't find a comfortable sleeping position, and as soon as I was at peace and fell asleep, Oleg needed to be fed again.

I ended up in a vicious cycle where everything revolved around the thought of my non-existent sleep, and I couldn't think or talk about anything other than sleep. I started off each week talking about how I would sleep during the coming weekend; Mike couldn't stand me anymore, he probably didn't understand the magnitude of my tremendous fatigue. Eventually, I didn't find anything enjoyable anymore; it felt like I was someone else, someone I didn't know. At my darkest moments I would be willing to sell our son in order to sleep and the next moment I felt sad and guilty because the thought had entered my head. Everyone at the Child Health Center assured me this was common. Oleg was gaining weight just as he should and it was normal to feel tired and lethargic. The nurse told me becoming a parent is a big adjustment and that it would all be fine. I really didn't feel normal in any way. The advice I got from the Child Health Center was that I should sleep during the day while Oleg slept, but I couldn't, even though I was so tired. It was because I had all of these things I needed to do, where did that come from? That, and the fact that I've never been able to lie down during the day and rest. I'm not that type. I finally lost it and burst into tears; all my energy and will were gone.

We sat down and started thinking about who would be able to help me.

We didn't have a big pool to choose from, so I wouldn't be able to get help that way; my parents still worked, and Mike's parents lived far away. We thought about siblings, friends, and neighbors. In the end, I decided to put up signs at a school and the grocery store, looking for a babysitter. It was so scary, to think that I would trust a stranger to take care of my child. I got a couple of answers and met two fifteen-year-old girls. They were both nice, so I decided that they would come to my house after school once a week to pick up Oleg and take him out in the stroller for a few hours.

It cost me seven dollars an hour, which was money well spent, since my anxiety subsided. Suddenly, I had two whole hours to myself. I didn't use that time to do anything specific; I usually just relaxed. It was the feeling of it, being able to read, take a shower, just be, that was so peaceful. I really longed for my "off" hours when I was with the baby, but after a couple of hours when he was gone, I started missing him again and ran back and forth between the windows, hoping to see the stroller.

Then what happened?

His first year, I regularly used the babysitters to take him for a walk.

Sometimes Oleg would be sleeping when the babysitter would arrive, so she would stay at home while I went out for a walk alone. One of the girls, Lisa, still works for us and Oleg has known her since he was a little baby, which is wonderful. He is turning three, so we usually get Lisa to work if we want an evening on our own to go to the movies or do something else. I don't understand why I felt so unsure and had such a guilty conscience for not taking him out on the walks myself.

New thoughts

Why am I so scared of asking for help when I don't know how to do something myself? When I tell others about what I had done, I have to face wrinkled brows, shaking heads, and questions about how I had the guts and why I did it.

It was about survival.

As a parent, it's important to have a functioning network, no matter what the situation is. If someone doesn't have a big network of family members, they can try to start a new network of neighbors, friends, colleagues, and helpers like paid babysitters, cleaners, purchasers, and launderers. At the same time, I would also like to help others. A system of bartering services would be great.

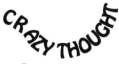

My milk—no thank you!

My four-week-old baby and I are crying. I barely have any milk coming from my breasts, it's light blue and thinner than tears. The nurse from the Child Health Center encourages me to breastfeed more and when I follow her advice, my son and I feel even more unhappy.

Nicole with Erick, age 5.

Erick is my firstborn, my one and only wonderful child. In my fifth month of pregnancy, I learned that my husband was having an affair with another woman. This was a betrayal, which of course made me very unhappy. I remember the first thought that came to my head was that I didn't want to have the child. I felt that it was going to be completely impossible to do this by myself, while I also realized that it was a fact that I was going to have a child. My husband moved out and I was on my own. We had been so happy that we were going to have a baby, but after all of this, I didn't look forward to having him at all.

I remember that I lived my life in a fog. I wasn't hungry and therefore barely ate. My husband moved back home as the birth of our child was approaching, so that he could be there for the arrival. It was a strange period of time and I found it hard to believe that he had ended the relationship with the other woman. I still found it impossible that we were having a child, whom we would look after and take care of together. It did happen though and once Erick was born it felt like everything had happened for a reason. I immediately fell in love with him and he became, besides simply my son, a consolation in all that had happened to me.

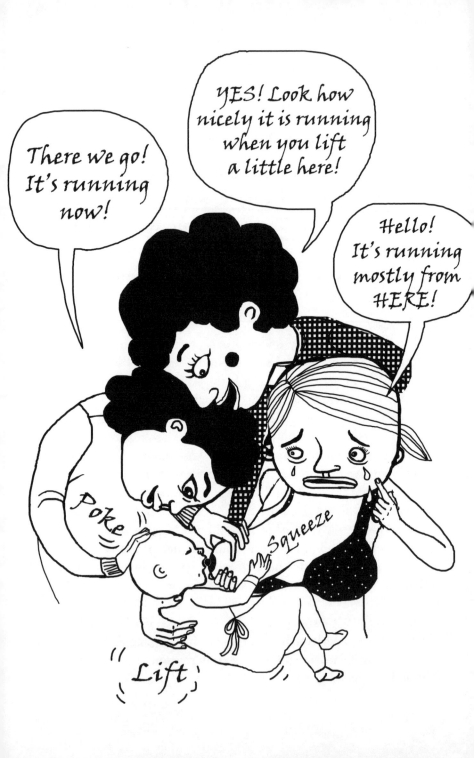

The breastfeeding was hell from the very beginning. Erick suckled and suckled but he was never satisfied.

I breastfed and breastfed and I was never happy. My milk was light blue and very thin. At the Child Health Center I was constantly told how the milk would come out if I continued to breastfeed Erick, and boy did I breastfeed. It was as if we were stuck together all day and all night. We continued like this for the longer part of my early parenthood, the nurses at the Child Health Center watched me while I breastfed. Couldn't they see that I was miserable? In retrospect, it's obvious that I couldn't nurture my baby with my own milk, as I hadn't eaten in weeks.

I had also read and heard about how healthy and gratifying it is to breastfeed your child. If I breastfed, he wouldn't get any allergies, I would quickly get in shape (what shape?) after the pregnancy, my uterus would quickly tighten, and most of all, it's so helpful to always have food with you—just at the right temperature and all. . . . Didn't I read somewhere that breastfeeding would make me calm and relaxed thanks to some hormone the body releases? Calm and relaxed? I was disappointed, tired, and so very unhappy. Where could I find the hormone that cured that? I also felt so terribly sorry for the little baby, my child, who I was responsible for taking care of and feeding, who remained sad and hungry.

I followed the advice that I had gotten at the Child Health Center, to breastfeed more, almost like a slave, for several weeks. At that time I didn't even consider not breastfeeding; it just wasn't an option. It wasn't just the people at the Child Health Center who paid a lot of attention to breastfeeding, everyone else had the "how is breastfeeding going?" question on the top of their list of topics they wanted to discuss.

One Friday night when Erick was four weeks old, we were invited to my sister's for dinner. When we got there, Erick wouldn't stop screaming and I had had enough. I went from sad to angry in a second and pretty much ordered Erick's father to run down to the convenience store to buy baby formula and a bottle. Despite my anger and resolve, clouds of anxiety quickly started to move in. What is going to happen to Erick now? Will he develop all sorts of allergies? Am I giving up too easily? Should I breastfeed a little more before I give up? What if it all works out tomorrow? The clouds had quickly passed, I had taken the decision and it was break or make it time. There was no room for regrets!

Erick's dad returned with a bottle and small carton of baby formula. I was so determined to do this that I quickly rinsed off the baby bottle, tore the carton open, and poured it into the bottle.

I placed it in the microwave and was about to throw the carton into the trash, when I glanced at the best-used-before date. The formula wasn't very fresh, but I just didn't care. I had made a major decision and didn't plan on changing my mind. I heated it all in the microwave to just the right temperature (something some microwaves are capable of, too!). I gave the kid the bottle—he suckled and was finally eating! My shoulders dropped down a couple of inches from my ears and I noticed that I was breathing, which was something I don't know if I had done for several months. I think my uterus might have contracted a tad, too.

Then what happened?

Erick slept all weekend after drinking that bottle. I bought more fresh formula and continued feeding him. I tried going back to breastfeeding for a while, but gave up pretty quickly. I still wasn't completely happy to be giving up on breastfeeding and the fact that Erick was full of formula. Erick's father and I still had issues, but I didn't have to struggle with my thoughts and feelings of not being able to feed my child. I couldn't get over what my husband had done when I was at my most vulnerable time in my life, and so we decided to go our separate ways.

Now and then, I wonder what effect stopping the breastfeeding so early might have on Erick. Especially since he has always had a rocky relationship with food. He doesn't eat much and prefers to only eat tortellini, but it's a consolation to see that he's happy and he's growing like he should.

New thoughts

Baby formula is good for children, too. It's nice to think for yourself and decide what you want to use! It's important as a parent to try and make things easier for yourself.

We don't need a parenting course

Parenting classes are available in most areas. It's a good idea, an offer that I can decline or accept, and a choice that I have to make as a prospective parent. But I don't feel that I have a choice. It's quite the opposite, as I feel that my partner and I have to attend. Neither of us wants or feels the desire to attend the course.

Emmy with Mark, 2 months.

I really didn't want to attend some silly course where I would have to share my expectations and feelings about childbirth and parenthood. It's really not my thing.

When I want to talk about it, I do it with my friends or my partner, not with a whole group of people I do not know, where our only common ground is that we will give birth around the same time. I want to decide for myself who I'll share my expectations, hopes, and fears with. My friend Sara told me about the time her brother and his wife attended the class for the first time and everyone was split into pairs to talk about equality in the relationship and at home. You weren't supposed to talk to your partner, but you were to discuss equality in the relationship with a complete stranger. But what does that mean?

It feels like a concept someone made up to pass time, talking about equality before you have any idea how it will all actually turn out. How are you supposed to know, or even speculate, about how things are going to be when the baby arrives. I just wanted to focus on the baby that was going to be coming out of me.

I met a girl at the Child Health Center when I was there for a diabetes test. She told me she took the class before and she thought it was really bad; they had to make silly diagrams of how much time they had before they had the baby, and how much time they would have after having it. How would you be able to know that?

No way, I thought. I can spend my time doing better things.

It's just not my thing. I would be happy attending lectures to learn more about breastfeeding or giving birth, but I don't want to be a part of one of those groups.

Our midwife nagged us for making the choice to not to attend the course. We received, without fail, little hints almost every time we went for a checkup. She tilted her head slightly to one side and said, "We discussed that in the last class . . . oh, that's right, you don't attend the course." Or when I asked a question, the answer was always followed by: "We talk a lot about that in the course."

I often felt that what we did was wrong. Our choice not to attend wasn't seen favorably, and they would let us know about it—not punish us, but let us know. My suspicions were proven correct when we started looking for a good maternity ward in our city. We were interested in visiting a place and we told our midwife at a checkup. But the midwife told us that visiting the maternity ward was part of the course and unfortunately, they could not offer any visits to those who chose not to partake. All we were allowed to see were pictures on the hospital's website to get the idea of what it looked like. We could also go online and look at a video of the maternity ward.

Then what happened?

Mark still arrived and everything worked out fine. Toward the end of the pregnancy I admit I was feeling a little stressed since I hadn't read a lot about giving birth, but it probably wouldn't have made a big difference for me anyway. The staff at the maternity ward was amazing and helped our uneducated selves as much as they could. It didn't really matter that we hadn't been there previously to have a look; we got all the help and guidance we needed once we were there.

New thoughts

Who should you attend a class for? I usually do it for myself and not because someone else thinks I should or must.

I also understand those who want to attend and who think that it's important, interesting, or just a nice way to prepare. They can do whatever they want. We didn't think we'd become worse parents or have a worse time during childbirth, it's just that the concept didn't work for us. Our midwife used the course as an instrument of control, and she constantly went on about it and told us about what we were missing. When I, as an individual, didn't do as she said during my pregnancy, I was in the wrong—according to her.

Not doing the "right" thing evokes feelings of doubt, and I wonder what's right and what's wrong.

Who decides?

We're not moving in together

We are in love, we are close to each other, we share our lives. But others still find it hard to understand that we don't want to live together.

Lisa with Beth, age 2.

During my pregnancy, Thomas and I decided that we would keep our respective homes and not move in together. We would figure out the practical aspects eventually, but I wanted to keep my apartment and Thomas wanted to keep his house in the suburbs for his older boys. I didn't even consider going out to the middle of nowhere with a small baby; it was important for me to be close to life and activity, and not have to depend on a car or the bus to go into the city.

We agreed that we would still spend a lot of time together and our baby would see us both as much as she needed. Only time would tell if we'd end up spending one week in the suburbs and one week in town. One of the first questions we were asked at the time of the enrollment at the Child Health Center was: Are you living together with the father of the child?

"Yes, we are together, but we don't live together."

Naturally, there were follow-up questions about how we would arrange everything, if we were going to move in together at some point, and how it would work in practice with a small baby. I really felt that we didn't fit into the existing framework; you are either with the father of the baby, which means that you live together, or you aren't together and you live apart. I was expecting that a lot of people would have opinions about not living together when you are sharing children and are still a couple, but I was not prepared for how everyone would freely speak of

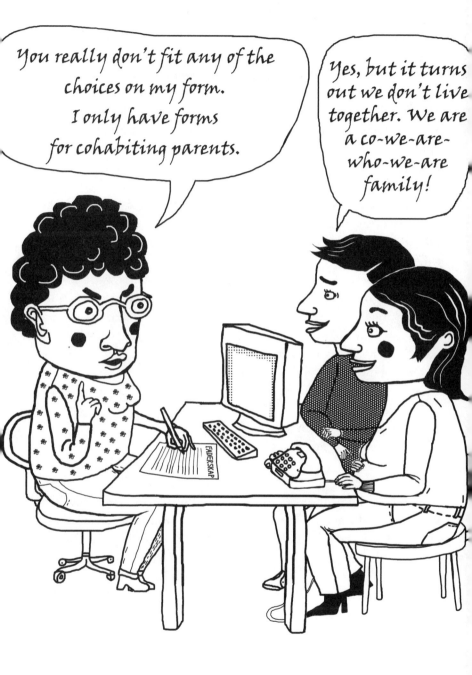

their prejudices about our relationship and if it was a good or bad thing to do. I think there's a bigger acceptance of alternative family dynamics in cities compared to smaller towns.

You're viewed as odd and deviant when you don't follow the norm. We're both a little older and we don't care about what others think, but I could see how it would be harder for someone who feels more anxious and insecure when others question their decisions. A funny story we tell is when we went to child support services to sign a paternity form. I wanted to do it before Beth was born to prevent any confusion if anything should happen to me during labor or during our first days. If I died, Thomas wouldn't have custody if there weren't any signed paternity papers. A lady at the child support services told me on the phone that this would not do! Everyone usually signs the paper after the birth of the baby! But I don't want to wait, I told her. I want to do it earlier, is that a problem? It wasn't really, the only tiny problem was that they don't usually operate that way. Doing things the usual way is always the right way, right?

The next shock for the child support services lady was when she asked for our address and I gave her two.

"Do you own two homes?"

"No, we live in separate places."

"But are you together?"

"Yes, we are very much together."

"So you have two addresses because of tax reasons?"

"No, that's not it."

We went on and on like this with a woman who did not want to accept that we had our separate homes, and I finally got tired of explaining, so I ended the conversation with "I'll see you next week!" When we arrived, she started off the conversation by saying that this isn't the way it usually happens. We listened as little as possible, leaning over the papers that we were supposed to sign, only to find one address filled in—Thomas's address. We had two separate addresses and we wanted both to be written down! The lady just thought we were weird and continued blabbering on about tax reasons and where is the baby going to live and are we really a couple. But we made her fill out a new form and then it was time to sign. As I read the document, I found a major mistake; she had written down the wrong year of the conception—when Beth was made—and according to this incredibly important document, which preferably should only include one address, I had been pregnant for a year and nine months. It had to be a new world record. But we signed anyway without saying anything, just because we thought it was hilarious.

Then what happened?

I wrote a very angry letter to the head of the office and received a personal response by phone. She asked if I wanted to take this further, but I thought her phoning me and having a conversation with our administrator was enough. I thought, so how are others treated, those without a partner or who are gay or are living in an entirely different way? Social Services is there for our sake, to provide the service and the support residents need. We are living in a new millennium and the cohabitating family is no longer the only norm.

New thoughts

No, other than the fact that my preconceptions of Social Services were confirmed. You need to be strong in order to be able to stand up for your opinions and thoughts and your way of living, especially if they are outside of the accepted norms of what a family should be or look like.

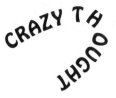

We can do it all!

When not just one but several of my favorite bands are playing a concert, is it assumed that I should stay home with our newborn baby? Both of us want to go. Could it work?

Anna with Sara, age 6, and Simon, age 12.

This was many years ago. Twelve to be exact. Time has passed quickly and it feels like it just as easily could have been yesterday. The festival was in full swing, and a lot of great rock bands were going to perform. With a newborn baby and two parents who were both interested in seeing the bands, the situation felt hopeless. For me, as a mother, that is. No matter how equal we tried to be, I was the only one breastfeeding. And Simon was one of those babies who wanted to eat a lot. Pumping my breast milk wasn't an option; I found it very difficult and could hardly manage to get anything out, and Simon couldn't figure out how to drink from a bottle. Having a babysitter was, therefore, not an option for us. So I sighed and prepared myself to be the one who missed the fun and would stay home.

Parenting was new and wonderful and I was so happy being a mom, but after two months, we gradually started to get into our routines. One day, when went for coffee in town and were walking with the stroller, I heard rock music echoing through the summer air, and I felt a stab— because of a desire that I was trying to repress. The desire to get out, experience something different, listen to music, and forget about sore nipples and diapers full of poo. Forget about being a mother and just be Anna for a while.

And perhaps that's how the idea came to me. I'm not sure who first uttered the words, but suddenly there they were. Why not try bringing Simon along so we both could go? I shook my head, but that craving quickly reappeared—the longing to actually go out as a family. It surely couldn't be impossible. We discussed it back and forth; Simon was, after all, an "easy" baby to bring along as long as one of us carried him in a baby carrier attached to the shoulders. He was usually comfortable and almost always fell asleep. But as new parents, we also felt uncertain. Could we really do this? Would we hurt him in any way? And the obvious: What would others think?

We talked objectively about it and came to the conclusion that the worst that could happen was that one (me) or both of us would have to go home. That would be that. Disappointing, but not much to do about it. He wouldn't go without food, as I always had it with me. We could change his diaper in the bathroom or on a patch of grass if it was an emergency, and there were bins everywhere. What about the sound, would he become deaf due to the high noise level? We bought earplugs at the pharmacy and grabbed the thickest hat we could find and pulled it down over his little ears. We were ready!

We took the train into town and walked with Simon strapped in the baby carrier on my shoulders. He blinked in wonder at the sunshine and all the people who were heading in the same direction. I cautiously glanced around. There were no strollers in sight. But we were here anyway, my little family, and we were going to have fun.

Once we got to the festival, we saw some of our friends. We talked a bit, walked around, and listened to the band that was playing on stage. It was loud, but we stayed toward the back.

We felt that we had a lot of eyes on us; people were glancing furtively. A baby at a rock concert? Are they completely crazy? I imagined that this was what they were thinking. We knew that our child was doing well, but did other people realize that? I felt exposed and I nearly wished that I had a sign that read: "This baby has earplugs and is doing great right now." Incredibly silly and totally unjustified! Who was singling me out to be a lousy and selfish mother, was it people around me or was it me?

When the band started playing and we found that Simon had fallen asleep, we relaxed and got the rock experience we were hoping for. He safely hung off my belly while we listened to the howling guitars. What we had been worrying about was all of a sudden easy and straightforward. We could take this little package anywhere!

As band number two started to play, Simon woke up and was hungry. Good timing, we thought, and walked off along the water and found a quiet spot on the grass. I sat there in peace and breastfed until Simon was full and happy. After we quickly changed his diapers, Matt took over and carried the baby; my back was sore and I was very sweaty.

That afternoon we got to see three bands. Simon slept two-thirds of the time and only woke up twice for food. It was an amazing experience and we felt even more proud. Our little two-month-old baby, in the middle of a music festival, rocked to sleep by rock music. We were really cool parents!

Then what happened?

I actually think that the trip to the concert made us better parents. Something as simple as bringing the baby to something that demonstrably wasn't the least bit complicated strengthened us tremendously. It also made us sure that we knew what was best for our children.

The next steps were small; we dared going to restaurants and traveled long distances. And naturally, we went to more festivals. We later told Simon that he attended his first rock concert when he was two months old, and he thinks that's really cool!

New thoughts

We can do most things with our children. They can come with us if we have the desire and energy. I've found that it's me, not anyone else, who sees problems where there are none, and that I—no matter how liberal I think I may be—am pretty controlled by social conventions. I do my best to ignore some of them. I don't care if others look down on me when I have my children with me at a bar or a concert or in any other so-called "adult" place. I am the one who knows my children the best and what is right for my family.

Dare to decline responsibility!

I'm the type of person who is a member of many boards, councils, planning groups, and committees. I always say yes when I am requested to be the spokesman (doing all the work, which others in the group can take the credit for when it's done). I am a permanent note-taker. I win "Father of the Year" every year. I have a hat that says COMPETENT on it. Responsible is my middle name.

Kat with Eric, age 4, Jasper, age 9, and Gustav, age 11.

I have, for most of my life, been a part of the Parents' Association and the Residents' Association. At the start, I actually enjoyed it . . . or hold on . . . it actually started with me feeling acknowledged and competent when I was asked—you are such a good writer, you are in the know, they listen to you . . .

This was when I was still in college and I now realize how long I've been doing this for. Talk about a habit! I haven't suffered, and at times, I really have enjoyed being the one who brings up issues, starts projects, and makes things happen. Yes, I can write, I am in the know, and people often listen to me, but just like with all labels, when is it ever fun being a stereotype? I don't always enjoy speaking for other people, taking the risk of being criticized for believing in something, and having less time for my family and myself!

A few years ago, I was lying in bed, thinking. I felt a lot of pressure and everything felt like an obligation. At the time I was a member of the kindergarten PTA, the board of the elementary school's Parents'

Association, and the Residential Association (how did I manage to get myself into all of this?). What particularly stressed me out that night was that I had taken it upon myself to take minutes at the parents' meeting that day.

In the dark, in my bed, and with a bit of anxiety, I start thinking of quitting. Since I like doing things differently, the thought excited me even more. I painted a picture in my head of what the scenario would be if I quit all my duties and, from then on and throughout the spring semester (this was early January), would not take a single note.

Bye-bye, Residents' Association! Bye-bye, PTA! When I second-guessed myself, I would tell myself: "It's important to let other parents have a go at it; having new boards is a good thing." I asked myself why I did all of these things in the first place and the answers made it easier for me to "break up" with all of these responsibilities.

As for the Residents' Association, I really don't know how I ended up there. I'm not interested at all in speed bumps, noise barriers, common land, or neighborhood coalitions (with all due respect to anyone who is). And then there was the kindergarten PTA. My God, I had been a member ever since it was created! Besides, wasn't I the one who started it? I also comforted myself with: "If I change my mind, I can always just rejoin."

When I arrived at the Parents' Association at school the next day, I decided that I actually wanted to stay. I started thinking about what was in it for me, and I realized that I enjoyed being a part of it. I liked the other parents on the board. I liked being able to influence my children's everyday lives. I liked knowing what was going on at school because it benefited my children. I realized that my reasons for being in the Parents' Association were rather egoistic before. It was all about my children and me, but it benefited other children and parents as well. I suddenly felt as if my involvement had been about appreciation; I was doing something that was good for my children, myself, and a whole lot of other people.

It was fairly easy to drop my positions on the boards, but I was still doing tasks like taking minutes and participating in the various group projects. I decided that I would have zero tolerance. I would just be a

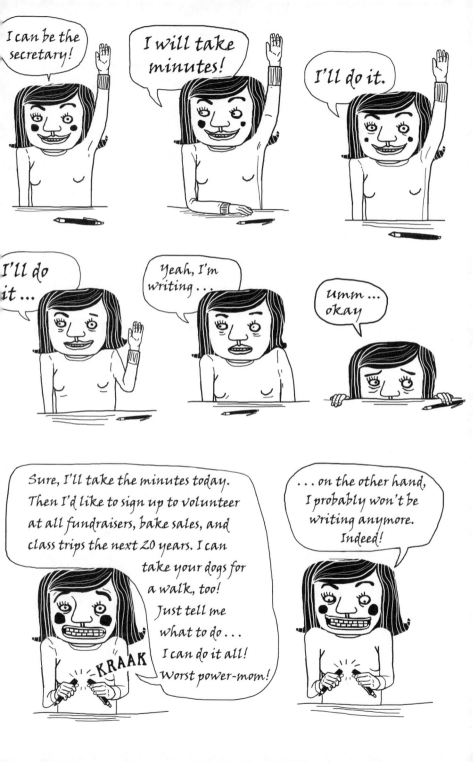

part of the school's Parents' Association and I would say no to all other things! In a way, it felt so mischievous and exciting that I would only do things that I wanted to do. I went around with a smile on my face and waited to share the news at the next meeting.

I finally received the invitation to the parents' meeting at my youngest son's school.

I motivated myself by thinking "come on, girl, you are going to have so much fun!" and off I went. Usually, I talk a lot with others and I often ask for help, but I hadn't done that this time. It felt like a big deal, and that it was mine, and I didn't want anyone but me to do this. I was with another mom who complained and said, "Now I'll be elected to some group that is going to arrange the garden party." You better believe it, I thought. You should join and I will come and enjoy it! Ha!

Once we sat down on the little chairs, the superintendent started off by saying: "Could someone possibly take notes during the meeting?"

I don't know how it happened. It took a millisecond until I heard someone slightly sigh and say, "I will."

The crazy part was that it was me speaking. When I realized this, my brain fired up. But, hold on . . . I'm not a minute taker . . . I've quit . . . or I am at least trying to cut back. I don't know how long it took but all of the sudden I had a pen and a paper in my hand and I heard words coming out of my mouth: "Look, the fact is that I am trying to quit taking minutes. So, I'm wondering who needs these," I said, waving the paper and pen.

At this point, some people started smiling and some were looking down at the floor with troubled faces. One of the dads offered to do the job. I know I didn't listen too much to what was said during that particular parents' meeting. I was mainly thinking about what was happening and whether it was good or bad. I concluded that it was positive, a little bit scary, and very fun.

This is going well, I thought, and I attended the next parents' meeting at school a few weeks later, cheerful and determined. The teacher at school had been inventive (and that should be commended), as she had taped a minute sheet and a pen underneath a chair in the classroom. She revealed this after we had sat down and all the parents nervously started groping underneath their chair. Guess what I found under mine? So, I did something that I didn't really think through. When a late parent was sneaking in through the door, I moved to another free chair—which only had graffiti and some old chewing gum on the underside.

This could have turned into a crazy situation, but it became amusing instead. The late parent didn't understand anything and took on the job, while I was recognized as funny and brave . . . (I left victorious, without taking any minutes, but with acknowledgment—my need for that is another story).

This is the way it continued but it usually wasn't as startling as the occasions I have told you about. Most of the time I just sat quietly—without looking down at the floor. One should be proud of following one's nose and needs! Before long, someone else took on the job.

Then what happened?

Right now I don't have any commitments. I'm not a part of the Parents' Association either. I very rarely take minutes. I think that's because I have written so many, it should be a while before I take on that mission again. I also think that much of what we do, when it comes to meetings/groups/documentations, is pretty unnecessary. I have concluded that schools, kindergartens, and associations don't stand or fall depending on me, and anyone can do what I do. If they get sick of it, they can say, "No thanks, I don't want to."

It's no big deal and I don't need to explain or excuse myself. I know what my responsibility is and I often ask myself: Is this my job? Do I want this? For whose sake am I doing this?

New thoughts

I am responsible for myself, my attitude, and my kids—period! However, I would like to share the difficulties that I wrestled with before I dealt with the issue and I think others struggle with. I leave here a small package of propositions, which you can open and use if you wish.

When you confuse musts with wants.

Remedy - make a map of your musts and go through them all. If they are in harmony with your wants, go ahead with them with pleasure and joy! If not, they go! You will need to remember to give yourself time to reconsider and reconcile. During that time, someone (who hasn't come as far in their development as you have) has probably accepted the task, while you didn't have to.

When you agree before you get the chance to think it through.

Remedy - to avoid habits, you need to remind yourself of what you are doing. This can be done with the help of an affirmation, for example: I take responsibility for what I want! I only do enjoyable things! I always give myself time to think! I'm really good at letting others work/delegate! I am learning something new!

Make your own one that speaks to you and remember that affirmations should be pleasing, uplifting, and expressed in the present tense (although it isn't actually true yet, you won't understand that you're being tricked).

Perhaps you'll be reminded by something in your pocket (like a photo of a minute taker crunched into a ball or a photo of a chairman that you painted a mustache, glasses, and pimples on). You can also ask people in your surroundings for help. You're not alone! There are other good people who can remind you when you are about to make the wrong decision.

Break everyday habits—and enjoy!

"Weekday all week long, bing bong!" sang a little girl to her mother each morning. Eventually this became their signature melody. They sang it every day, Monday through Friday. Weekdays didn't seem so bad after all, did they? With a little "bing bong," it was all right!

Our children's upbringing and our life consists of ordinary weekdays, so why not try to make it as easy and enjoyable as possible. Sometimes it may be tough, gray, and dull. That's how life is—like an eternal wave, it needs to go up as well as down. If it turns into one long gray line, we're probably not really living anymore. So let it rise and let it fall and don't let everyday life become one long boring trek toward the beckoning weekend.

Trying to find the simplicity of everyday life and not complicating it is easy to write about but harder to do, we know. But it should be nice being a parent and having a family should be fun—for the most part. One father described it this way: "The kid stands there, every day. She exists! Most days I love being a father, other days I think it's okay, and some days it's just about surviving."

Think of the artist who goes from painting nice and self-explanatory pictures, to a more vague and simpler style. Most might not understand what he is painting anymore, but the artist knows, and that's enough. He has found the simplicity. Parenting can be the same when parents have the courage to break patterns and norms that originally weren't even their own. To be able to diminish traditional parenting conventions, find your most manageable path, which might not be the easiest path for other people. It's brave, strong, and feels great.

Imagine that you're holding your toothbrush and it's time to brush your teeth. Where do you start brushing? Where did you start this morning and yesterday? What is it that makes you start to brush your teeth in the same spot every day? Okay, you might start brushing in different places each time, sure, that's great, but most of us start at the same spot every day. This is a pattern; it's something you do without really thinking about how, why, and if you want to change it. What would make you want to change this habit? Change is difficult, so we have to think, reflect, and sometimes stop for a second in order to avoid falling back into the same rut again. Patterns are repeated procedures that are located in our spinal cords; they exist in order to facilitate our everyday family lives and make the not-so-fun parts of our parenting easier. Routines help us to save energy, leaving room for what's enjoyable. You might be too tired to change because it takes too much energy at that moment.

When you think of someone as "experienced," it's usually someone who knows what she is doing and doesn't need to spend tons of time on things. If we go back to the knowledge stairs concept at the beginning of the book, it's like standing on the *unconscious knowledge* step, where you do things without having to think too much about it. Routines aren't just about putting the children to bed, feeding, and bathing them. A recurring routine is Christmas, for example. We do the same things every year, eat the same food, and place the tree in the same place. Shame on an adult who breaks the holiday traditions! There is an assurance in knowing that things stay the same, which is something that children and adults actually want and need.

We have spoken positively and happily about routines because they hold high value; they save our strength and energy for improvisation and joy. What does that have to do with breaking habits? Sometimes we are stuck in a habit of bedtime routines, sleep routines, or food routines that don't really work. Everything is topsy-turvy, but we hold on to those routines like an old, punctured inflatable circle that's barely floating on the water. Because we have to have our routines! They don't work, but we continue. Who says that we can't change our habits and do something completely new, something different? This is always a recurring thing with parents we meet—they do things a certain way but their routines aren't producing the results they want.

If we tell you that routines and habits will save you time and energy, you can ask yourself the question: Do they really, or am I caught up in something that I built up and that worked only before, or with the other children, or with the Smith family across the street? We are often our own biggest enemy when it comes to breaking patterns. The game of wrestling that we play with ourselves can be arduous. We may know that we need to change, but how, when, and why is it necessary to go against your habits? It's only you who can answer these! Think of how exciting it is when you start a new job and are still unfamiliar with the new place. You notice issues and problems that the old-timers don't anymore. It's the same when we want to break free from habits and routines at home—we need to become more aware of the problems they are causing.

When it comes to parenting and family, there are many unwritten rules on how things should or shouldn't be done. A lot of it comes from the common parental walls. It's as if some almighty God of parenthood decided what the wallpaper should look like. We may encounter resistance when we don't do what we "should." We step outside of the norm that others have made up and it can be hard to fight others' resistance, especially if you're not sure yourself if what you did was right. But the goal must nonetheless be to enjoy this string of days that's called everyday life as much as possible.

Breaking patterns can sometimes be about trying something new, doing it differently, but then going back to the old way because it was quite simply the best way. What often happens is that we feel satisfied and happy that our original way was the best. "I was doing the right thing from the beginning, I just needed to realize it myself," one mother told us. You break a habit for your own sake, not for anyone else's. But the clever part is that when you include your children in it, maybe even ask them for help, it becomes something that you do together. Our children, as well as ourselves, benefit from doing new things together, because in order to do something new, you need to be aware and present in what you are doing. To do something together, to change, can turn into an adventure, a game where everyone is included. It's a win-win for the parents and the kids! "Crazy as hell can be really enjoyable!" said one mother who we interviewed for this book, when she was about to go home and try out some new sleeping routines after being inspired by another parent who did something new at bedtime.

Sometimes, things turn out right when we make mistakes! With that motto, we'll have the courage to try, to play, and to laugh at ourselves and the hilarious parts of being a parent.

One attempt can be enough, and it might just be the deal breaker that makes us get out of something that isn't working for us in everyday life. When we do crazy things, our children join in on the fun, and later, you can reminisce about your crazy adventures. "Remember when we slept in our tent in the living room? Remember when we ate dinner on the balcony in the middle of winter?" Remembering together means being together.

Our shared memories live on for a long, long time. We leave an imprint with our children and they make an imprint on us, and that's the way it should be. Be sure of yourself, trust yourself, be brave, have fun—because it's all worth it.

What do you need to start doing in order to make your everyday life more enjoyable?

What do you need to stop doing in order to make your everyday life more enjoyable?

What do you need to do more of in order to have fun as a parent?

What do you need to do less of to have fun as a parent?

When should you do it?

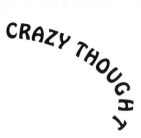

Finders keepers!

One might at times think that my children were adopted. Our interests are totally different; as a parent, I want things to be happening all the time and think it's boring to do nothing and putter around.

Helena with Malin, age 5, and Patrick, age 7.

Sometimes I got so tired of my kids—the same old whining, same fights, and dull questioning. They weren't very fun or particularly cute and neither was I for that matter, and I sounded like an old record player. We started at point A, went around point B, reached point C, and then we were back at A again. I was fed up with myself and really fed up with my two whiners. We were really stuck in a boring routine. Our weekends were proof of all the dullness and pestering. We used to do a lot of fun things— we went to the movies, went on trips, watched television, went out for ice cream. I, at least, felt that we did enjoyable and fun things together, and it was important to me that we had active weekends, but later, all I had to do was come up with a suggestion for an activity and the complaining would start: "No, not a trip, I can't be bothered sitting in the car for a long time"; "It's a boring idea, I don't feel like it"; "I want to stay home."

They had become two miserable teenagers who completely dismissed James and me and our ideas. I'd always get upset and say something like: "Okay then, we'll stay home and have a boring time, if that's what you want." What frustrated me the most was that I was the only one who wanted to do things and not just stay at home. James felt completely satisfied with staying at home and so did the kids. I complained a lot to my friends and coworkers about how boring my children were and how they sometimes drove me completely crazy by not wanting to do anything.

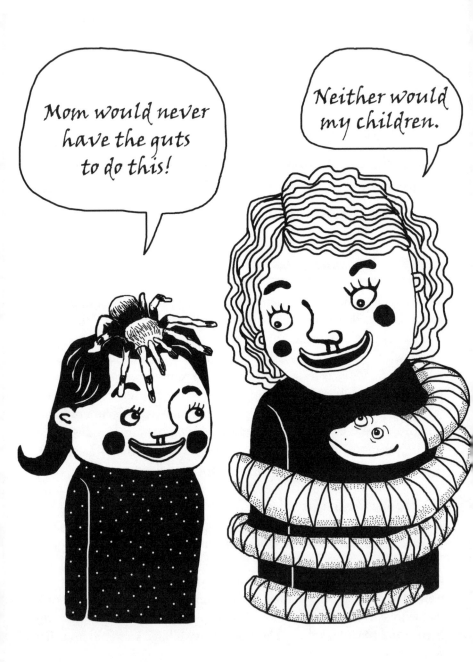

My colleague, Karin, felt that I should be happy that my children liked being at home since she had two kids who always complained about them never doing anything fun together. Karin didn't have the energy to do anything else other than stay at home on weekends. She enjoyed doing crafts around the house, painting pots, baking, and all the things that make me cringe.

"I don't want to go anywhere or schedule things on the weekends, I want to be off," said Karin.

"Maybe we should swap children," I laughed and Karin agreed, and that was that. But the following weekend I felt that I really would like to swap children, as there was a pet exhibition that I wanted to bring Malin and her friend to, but Malin preferred playing at Ida's house to going to a boring exhibition that she could attend another time. I asked Patrick to come, but he wanted to be with his father and paint something in the garage. So there I was, alone and annoyed. I called Karin and asked her if I could borrow her girls and bring them to the pet show, and learned that they really wanted to go. Karin was beaming. Said and done, I had two new children and they were miracles of kindness and positive feelings. They thought the show was great fun and talked incessantly about the animals—which ones were the cutest, softest, and the most fun.

We had a really nice afternoon and they were super excited when I returned them to their real mother. My own children had barely noticed that I was gone. This became a tradition and we swapped children periodically. Karin likes crafts, so when she'd bake, paint pots, or make candles, she'd invite my children over. They enjoyed these indoor activities and she was incredibly patient with the kids, which is a talent I don't have.

Whenever I'd suggest an activity and my children didn't want to do it, I called Emma and Marie, who enjoyed doing things with me. So far it's only been for one day at a time, but why wouldn't we be able to swap children for a whole weekend? My kids are happy and nice when they are with Karin and her girls are really fun to do things with. I have also noticed that my kids like doing things with me whenever Karin's girls are around; they enjoy other children and I think it makes a difference that Emma and Marie are so happy to be with me. Sometimes the four of them will be with me and other times they are with Karin.

Then what happened?

We have continued with our children swapping. I like her girls and she likes my whiners, who aren't whining when they're with Karin. We usually joke about our children having two families and we wonder where they really want to live. Sometimes I feel that Karin's girls are more similar to me than my own children are, especially when it comes to interests. I love my children to death and I know that they love me, but I like meaning something to others who really show their appreciation for the things I plan. Karin's oldest girl Emma is nine years old, and she will at times call me herself and ask if I want to take her to the swimming pool or the museum. It feels great that she sees me as an adult friend who she is brave enough to call and talk to.

New thoughts

My own children presume that I'll always be there. We take each other for granted and there is something safe about that, but at the same time, it's easy to fall into boring routines and not appreciate each other for who we are. I think that's common in all relationships, whether it be our children or a partner. I also have to accept that we are different and have different interests. I'm not the only one who gets to do things my way, which is sad but true. That's probably what made me feel so frustrated, nobody wanted the same things as me. What makes me feel a little bitter, a little envious even, is that if Karin comes up with a suggestion, it's almost always welcomed, but if I suggest something, there are always some complaints. But maybe that's just me being childish.

I've also been thinking about my own childhood, when my mom and dad almost every weekend forced me and my siblings to go with them to auctions and antique stores. To this day I hate old stuff and wouldn't even attend an auction if someone paid me. Their interests became a family affair and we could never say no. I'm glad that my children can speak up and know what they want; that's important.

Neighborhood watch with Auntie Berg

I'm exhausted as soon I get inside the front door with the children, the shopping bags, various gadgets, and the mail. I'm thinking that it should be at this time that I would want to cuddle with my children, read books with them, and let them tell me about their day, while I just watch them and listen. But instead I am thinking that I can't be bothered now—leave me alone!

Tina with Yvette, age 3, and Maya, age 6.

I often think about how important it is that my children feel they are being heard and appreciated, but at the same time, I find that I can't give that to them at certain times. It's common that when I want to be left alone, that's when they need me the most. Although I admit that I second guess whether they really need me when I think they do, but I assume so.

This usually happened when I'd pick them up from daycare. It made me happy to see them on the playground, but getting their things together to leave always turned into so much work that the joy kind of disappeared. I often had to rush from work to daycare, then spent lots of time looking for a missing sock, mitten, sweater, or drawing, and struggled to get the kids home. Getting the kids into the car usually went smoothly, and I'd feel relieved to have them and their things all ready to go in the car with me. Then came the unloading outside the house, which didn't go as smoothly. They would fight about which side of the car to get out of, they don't want to help carry things, or the worst possible scenario: they wanted to be carried into the house.

On the way to the front door I'd take the chance to reach in the mailbox, shoving envelopes under my armpit or in my mouth. How I managed to find the keys and unlock the door, I can't even describe, it's just something that happened. Then my tired, usually frowning and dirty children and a totally exhausted mom/pack mule stumbled into the hall, where hungry cats and a crazy dog greeted us. It was all too much!

This was the time that I felt bad for not giving my kids enough attention. I just wanted to be left alone! Then one day, when all the things I just mentioned had happened, and I was parking in the driveway, the girls asked if they could go to Sonja's house. Sonja is our wonderful neighbor the girls call "Auntie Berg," but usually we only visited her on the weekends. At first, I said no. I was sure Sonja wanted to be left alone on a weekday like this, and the point was that you "should" be with your children during the short period between daycare and bedtime. But I quickly succumbed to their pleas and dropped the girls off at Sonja's.

This was when my new life began. Calmly I carried in the bags and groceries and got the mail. The house was quiet. I petted the dog, fed the cats, sorted through all the things that I brought with me, read the mail, went to the bathroom, unpacked my work bag, then went on the computer and read through my emails. I was calm and systematic as I wandered about, because I really enjoyed it. I thought about everything and nothing, it was like meditating. This would take me about a half hour and after, Maja would come through the door and I was so happy! We cuddled for a while, talking, listening, and enjoying each other's company. Then Yvette would come and again I was so happy! We cuddled too until she wanted to do something else. The whole evening was different. I wasn't even annoyed that the girls barely ate their dinner because they were full from all the cookies they ate at Sonja's.

Then what happened?

They don't go to Sonja's every day, but almost. She hasn't complained about the 4:30 PM visits. We have changed the routine somewhat by making the girls carry their stuff into the house and take off their coats first. I don't want Sonja to have to deal with all the dirty coats and shoes. The girls are happy to help with carrying things in because they know it's mandatory if they want to go visit her. I've also started telling the girls that they are only allowed one cookie each, so that they have an appetite when they get home. Sometimes they eat one cookie each and other times they eat more, but they still eat dinner to show that the cookies didn't spoil their appetite.

New thoughts

I've thought a lot about why the kids choose to go to Sonja's as soon as they get back home after a long day at daycare. Could it be that they actually don't need me at this time? Could it be that they also felt that our homecomings had been really hard and that we solved the problem this way?

I have come to the conclusion that it's probably me who has an unfulfilled need in these situations. I need some downtime when I get home. I need to wind down after work and slowly transition into the evening.

It's nice that my children and neighbor help me satisfy that need.

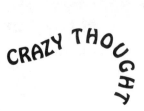

The daily puzzle that solves itself

Every time my husband and I look at the calendar on Sunday evenings, we get really frustrated. We twist and turn the pieces to prepare for the daily puzzle of the upcoming week—our lives—but there are too many pieces. We see that we are supposed to go to a parents' meeting, attend a soccer game and watch karate, and take the kids to swimming class on Wednesday in the space of two hours (and we mean the same two hours). How are we, two people, supposed to be in four places at once? Who is able to plan something like that? Not us!

Åse with Milla, age 4, Hedda, age 6, Tom, age 11, Karl, age 12, and Hampus, age 15.

I have a planning Nazi living inside me and I've always liked to plan, make lists, and complete things. It may sound dull, but it can actually be a lot of fun to plan things. In my planning I can also dream and envision how things will pan out.

Somewhere along the way, I can't remember when, the planning stopped being fun. I think it started being hard when I had three children. I remember how silly I thought I had been to feel that there was a lot of planning with the first child. It did, however, remind me that you

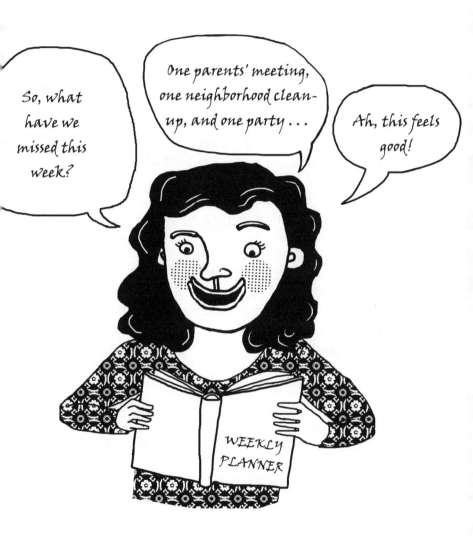

can't live life backwards and that there actually was a lot of planning during that period too, with one child.

With four children the coordinating started getting really hard, and the planning was at a very high and advanced level.

In our house, my husband Anders and I have different responsibilities. I do the laundry and am boss when it comes to everyday life, which we call the "connection center": I keep an eye on the details concerning the children during the week, writes notes for kindergarten and school, organize parties, and so on. Anders takes care of everything when it comes to feeding the family. He plans, buys, and cooks the food. When I think about it, everything is very divided in our home. We also find it hard to do each other's tasks. If Anders is going away somewhere and I have to cook, I'll make the fish sticks that Anders stocks the pantry with, because it's pretty much the only thing I can cook—unless I order takeout. If I'm away, the laundry and other daily chores will stand still, and they all must fend for themselves as well as they can. We can't keep track of each other's territory, nor do I have the energy to learn how to do something new.

When we had more children, there was obviously more food shopping and cooking and more laundry to do. It was working fine and wasn't a ton of more work . . . but I was becoming overwhelmed at the connection center! I couldn't have imagined how many activities there would be. It wasn't too bad until the kids grew up a little and started kindergarten. That's when it became so overwhelming that we decided to share the connection center tasks. I would still be the boss, but Anders would help me to come up with the game plan. I wonder how much time we have spent trying to plan impossible things.

In order to make sure that the planning would work, we had to coordinate everything with outside resources, often in the form of grandparents. It took so much time and yet we still weren't able to work it all out. Then one spring, during the most hectic time of our family life, it all fell apart. I reached a point when I just felt that the whole thing was too crazy. No matter how much I struggled with the planning, it went straight to hell. Everyone was always in the wrong place, the kids brought lunch with them on the wrong days (or more often on the right day, but a week too early), we missed parties, you name it. Everything just went wrong (it can be really hard remembering to put fruit in the lunch bags in the mornings; fruit can be pure hell).

We reached a turning point when we were supposed to bring two big cartons of ice cream in the morning for one of the kid's birthday celebrations at kindergarten so they could have it in the afternoon. Anders bought the ice cream and my responsibility was to bring it to the school and give it to the staff. So I did. In the afternoon, when I came to pick up the kids, I asked the teacher how the party went. She replied that it went well, but that "There wasn't much ice cream because the cartons were almost empty." At that point I started having a meltdown. I, the fool I was, took out two almost empty cartons of ice cream from the freezer, instead of the unopened ones. It was all too much for me! I was failing at everything! That's when it happened; I open my mouth and the most improbable story came out. The teacher looked at me, incredulous, then with an amused expression after I lied, "No, not again! This isn't the first time we've bought half-empty ice cream from the grocery store. I am so pissed off! I can't believe this is happening again and it's so typical that I brought these specific packages to kindergarten!"

After that I rounded up the kids and rushed home with flushed cheeks. How stupid can one be? I told Anders, who also thought that was really embarrassing. I argued a little and tried to get Anders to tell the kindergarten teacher the truth, but he didn't want to. I had to sort that out myself. I actually don't remember if I told the truth or if I made another story up. Looking back on it, it's all a fog. Ms. Monica from kindergarten, if I haven't apologized earlier for my strange lie, I'm sorry. I had to lie to save myself. I made too many mistakes in a short period of time and I couldn't bear it. Sorry!

My outlook changed after this incident. It's not possible to have a close eye on everything that goes on in a family of seven people. That daily puzzle that consists of a thousand pieces is impossible to do on Sunday evenings. We stopped trying. We went on with our lives and figured the rest would just have to work itself out. It was a brave thing to do, before I knew that things would indeed work themselves out. Once Wednesday rolls around, the sky clears up, a match will be cancelled,

Anders will go to the parents' meeting, I attend the karate class, and another parent takes the kids to swim class. This is when I'm glad that I haven't spent several hours trying to plan everything.

Then what happened?

There have been no more embarrassing lies in order to save my tail (only a few less embarrassing ones). These days I check the calendar every now and then to have an idea of what the week will bring. I am confident that things will work out. Sometimes things don't work out perfectly, but so what . . . ? Most times everything turns out fine. Everyone takes more or less responsibility to make sure things get done. We get a lot of spontaneous help from other parents and we gladly help others to solve their puzzles. It also makes me happy every time someone asks me whether it takes a lot of planning when you have a lot of children and I answer that we don't actually plan things.

A lot of people think it's crazy. Crazy or not, it works well for us.

New thoughts

Things often take care of themselves, if you let them. To fix things is great—to give up and stop trying is even better (sometimes).

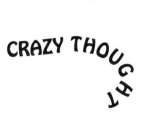

Not without my headphones!

I yell at my kids. More out of habit than frustration and anger. My children's bickering triggers me. Yes, simply that they make noise.

Peter with James, age 3, Sarah, age 6, and Lindsey, age 8.
I was a little older when Eva and I had our first child. I was very fascinated by my daughter and parenthood, and it didn't take long until we decided that we wanted another baby. Stupidly enough I believed that the baby would be a copy of Lindsey, and then Sarah appeared. It was crazy how interesting it all was and we knew that we wanted to do it a third time. I had a feeling that something new and unique was on its way. It was and when James came along, we had a set of unique and fun children.

Even though parenthood was a lot of work, it was all going pretty smoothly. Until one summer, when something changed. Sarah went from being a pretty quiet girl to being a girl who expressed all of her feelings, loud and clear. I had recently been thinking a lot about the fact that our oldest child had made me enter a new phase of my parenting. With Lindsey, I felt that I didn't "solely" need to be a caring father. I could be a person who could discuss things with my child and get something out of it on an adult level. I really enjoyed this new phase that I hadn't thought about before. I enjoyed being a parent even more. I was able to focus less on the nurturing, which meant that I had energy left over to try to understand Sarah. She shouted,

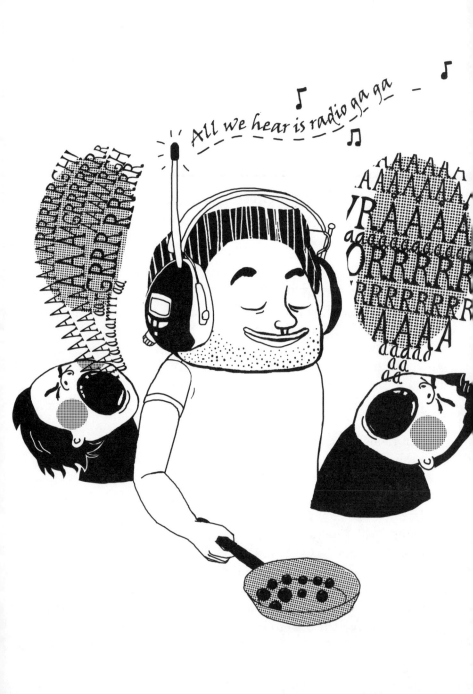

yelled, and fought and both Eva and I faced our up-until-now biggest challenge as parents. Our entire family became rougher and wilder in some ways.

I also started sounding off, loudly and clearly. Sarah's new behavior made us all louder, which was pretty easy to understand. You had to be heard, seen, and take up space. At the same time, Eva and I were happy that Sarah expressed her feelings, because we had been a little worried about the fact that it was sometimes difficult to understand what she was feeling before. I remember that we talked to her about why she didn't answer when someone asked her things. We didn't think she was shy. When we asked Sarah, she just told us that she did respond. We interpreted it as though she probably did, but that it was something that happened in her head. We found the solution when we actually assumed that she replied. Okay, we understand, you're telling us quietly inside your head. It allowed us to explain to her that she sometimes had to say things out loud so that she could be heard. We would remind her and that would be enough. Parenthood can be mercurial and time can pass by so fast. We went from having a child who mostly spoke in her head to suddenly having a child who expressed every single thought. At times, in a manner that wasn't always acceptable. This called for more effort on my part. I felt that it was important not only to point out what was acceptable, but also to actually demonstrate how to do things when trying to communicate something.

But acting on an idea can be difficult. Life goes on and you forget to do things. Without even noticing, I became a father who nagged, lectured, and yelled a whole lot at my kids. It didn't feel good. I wanted to be an attentive father who put energy into understanding my children. I wanted to be an adult. I was so incredibly sick of myself. More of myself than I was of my children who made a lot of noise. I got stuck in a routine that I wanted to break. Was there any relevance whatsoever in how I sounded? How would I be able to change?

One day, when I was making dinner, as usual, and the kids bickered, as usual, I heard myself ranting, nagging, and lecturing for the thousandth time. In that moment, I got an idea. I left the kitchen and got my headphones that I use at work. They're the kind that cover your ears and then some, and have a built-in radio. The kids didn't notice what was happening. I turned to a smooth rock station. At first it felt so good to block out the noise, and since I stood with my back facing the children, I couldn't see what they were doing. I was completely cut off. There was nothing that could annoy me other than the spaghetti and meatballs, and those things didn't really bother me.

After a while, I felt that there was silence behind my back. I imagined that the kids had stopped to think about what was different. "Something has happened—he's not making any noise." At that moment I was very aware of what I was doing and what might be happening behind my back. After a while I heard how they shouted at me, but I chose to pretend that I couldn't hear anything. Then one of the children came up to me and started to pull the leg of my pants a little. It wasn't until then that I loosened the headphones a little to ask my child what was wrong. It was nothing; when they realized that I was there, even though I didn't make any noise, they continued with what they were doing. That dinner was quite different. There was a peacefulness and harmony that I hadn't experienced in a long time.

Then what happened?

I felt that I used the headphones in order to break the pattern that I was very sick of. When I stopped interfering in the children's bickering, it was easier for them to find their roles and have functioning interactions with each other. I have used the headphones on a couple of other occasions. It has worked sometimes and other times the children took the opportunity to do something mischievous. But the headphones were mostly for myself and my habits that I wanted to break, and I think that happened the first time I put the headphones on.

New thoughts

It's not your fault that four people bicker. Doing something new and different can be the solution to breaking a pattern. To get rid of the trigger and cut the sound off by using headphones is ingenious!

My children are good at interacting with each other without me interfering every time. Sometimes it gets very loud though.

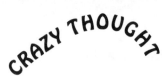

A dab or a toothbrush?

My children don't want to brush their teeth and the battle gets harder every day. Who says that you have to brush your teeth in the morning and evening? Is it the books about cavities that have left a lasting impression on us, or is it little Aunt Fluoride who sits on my shoulder and gives me a guilty conscience? I'm exhausted, and most of all, I want to punch Aunt Fluoride.

Carina with Lea, age 4, Mia, age 6, and Jasper, age 8.
We have been at war with all three of our children about brushing their teeth. It's been impossible to get this simple little routine to work. We've had battles every morning and every night, and if one of the children happens to object, we know that the other two will be even more difficult to handle. We may have had a really nice evening together, but as soon as the toothbrush comes out, the war begins. There is screaming and yelling and crawling on the floor in order to flee the toothbrush and the small amount of toothpaste. Sweaty, tired parents and angry, sad children were a normal sight in our home. The struggle started as soon as we said the magic word, brush . . .

Johan and I had given much thought to what the problem was; mass psychosis was one theory. Jasper had set the bar for what the others thought of brushing, as he was the oldest one. Another theory was that the brushing was associated with going to bed, which was the actual problem. We have put so much effort and energy into this big problem.

We have tried different solutions, from jointly holding one child at a time and force-brushing (which felt like physical and mental abuse for both parent and child), to long nagging sessions that end up with a fight, to reward systems with a gift after brushing ten times. It worked well until one of the angels freaked out and didn't want to play anymore. That's when total anarchy would erupt and the kids ran around, yelling and refusing to brush. We have brushed in the bathroom, in front of the TV, in bed, but nothing worked on our children. It was such a loaded subject in our house and I felt so much tension that I started to prepare myself after dinner for that night's imminent fight. When I tried to discuss a better way of handling the situation with our dentist, I don't think she listened, because she probably didn't understand what a huge problem this was for me, and probably because I tried to make it out to be less of a problem than it really was, to not seem foolish!

I talked to their teachers who thought it was terrible that my children refused to brush their teeth; thanks for hitting me when I'm already down. I'd never ask them for advice again. One morning I had had enough. I was so tired of these tooth-brushing fights and there was always a fight before we went to work, daycare, and school. They were, as usual, prepared for battle when I grabbed the toothpaste and told them about my new rules. In the morning, you could choose whether you wanted to suck on a dab of toothpaste or brush, but in the evening you had to brush.

Three little fingers appeared in front of me, and all of the children put the toothpaste in their mouths and everything was fine.

What a morning, I was absolutely euphoric when I got to work and I called Johan and told him about my new tactic. He was happy for me, but wasn't too convinced it was the right thing to do until he had time to think about it. He was all about things being right and wrong—what if the kids get loads of cavities, what will the dentist say, what will others say—but at the time I didn't care because I had managed to get through a difficult situation.

We went back to the dentist after trying out the new system. When she asked the children and me how the brushing was going, we were honest and said that we used dabs of it instead, once a day. I don't think she loved the idea, but we were certain in our belief, which was that this was the right way to deal with it at the time. We told her that when we brushed, we did it according to all the rules of brushing. After that she had a long monologue about the importance of avoiding sugar and corrosive substances, so she was more anti-sugar than anti-dabbing at that moment, which was nice for a mother who really tries to be good.

Then what happened?

We have continued doing this. They have to brush their teeth once a day and get a dab the other times. Sometimes they get to choose whether to dab in the morning or evening, but if they have had sweets during the day, they have to brush their teeth at night. The question in the morning in the bathroom therefore is: "A dab or a toothbrush?"

If they choose a dab, fingers will always appear, but one of them always tries to negotiate: If I choose the toothbrush now, will I get a dab tonight? It works well and I have to point out that none of the children have had cavities. We've actually asked a neighbor who is a dentist, if it makes a big difference to my children's teeth that they don't brush twice a day, but she doesn't think it does. So I've really thought our solution through, because I want to do the right thing.

New thoughts

I have suggested this solution to other parents who have told me about their toothbrush fights and I have been met with different reactions: "Is it possible?" "Don't the kids get cavities?" "How are you allowing this?" As if I was a bad parent! But I'm a great parent. In the fight over the toothbrush, we have found a solution that works for us, but it's not for everyone. We save a lot of energy that we can use for other things instead. I want Aunt Fluoride to know that I carefully watch what they eat when it comes to sugar and food that will corrode their teeth.

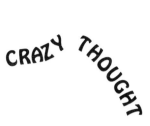
CRAZY THOUGHT

Silence is golden

I'm stuck in a sluggish goo of words, discussions, and communication. Will doesn't buy my explanations anymore, but does his own thing his own way. My patience is tested to the breaking point and anyone who knows him well can see how furious he gets.

Sofia with Will, age 4, and a baby on the way.
I have sometimes honestly felt that it's useless being a mom. It feels like a lifelong exam with no end in sight, and although I have a positive outlook on learning from the challenges that being a mother brings, it's the biggest and toughest thing I have done. It means feeling highs and lows, it's dynamic, amazing, and sometimes frustrating. As soon as you learn one routine, you lose it again; this is what I experienced the first years after having Will. I felt that I lost a part of myself, as I didn't have a balance between who I was, my job, my family, and being a mother. But as Will has grown older, it has been much better and I have also been able to use the aspects of my profession with him that I'm really good at, which is communication.

We talk a lot with each other, we are very communicative, we explain, verbalize thoughts and feelings, but sometimes it becomes too much. However, since communication is my best tool at work, I also have to use it at home. But there is a difference between using communication professionally and using it with my stubborn, sometimes angry son. Especially when I also get angry, because he knows which buttons to push to get to me, which would never happen at work.

For a period of time, it didn't matter what I said or did.

For two or three weeks, he opposed everything and the only answer I got when I spoke was "Bite me!"

"Put your jacket on if we are going to go out."

"Bite me!"

"Then we'll have to stay inside."

"Bite me!"

I got stuck in a communication trap and I tried explaining to him why one shouldn't talk like that—it made me sad and it was bad—nagging and information mixed together. As if Will cared at that point! He was just angry and was testing my limts; how far could he take it before I couldn't take it anymore?

I finally asked a friend for advice and he told me that he was silent in situations like that. He told his child that there was no point in talking when he was being nasty, and asked him to come back when he felt better and they would talk. When his child calmed down and approached him, they could continue talking, but until then, silence prevailed.

This was really difficult for me, as I am used to talking about everything. But I tried it the next time we had a fight. I said I thought it was nasty when he said "Bite me" and that I felt sad and that I wasn't going to talk to him when he behaved like this and used bad words when talking to me.

This was completely new to Will. He tried to get my attention for a while. He went "Mom, Mooooom, Mom" for a long time, but when he realized that I was serious and that I wasn't going to give in, he came to me and told me that he would stop.

Then what happened?

I'll still use this technique sometimes when we get into disputes, but I always tell him why I'm not going to fight with him. And then I have to hold out until he comes to me.

Our big fights, especially the nasty ones, have been occurring less frequently and are easier to handle.

The result is that Will uses it against me too, especially when he's angry or mad at me. He also says that he isn't going to talk to me because he's mad at me.

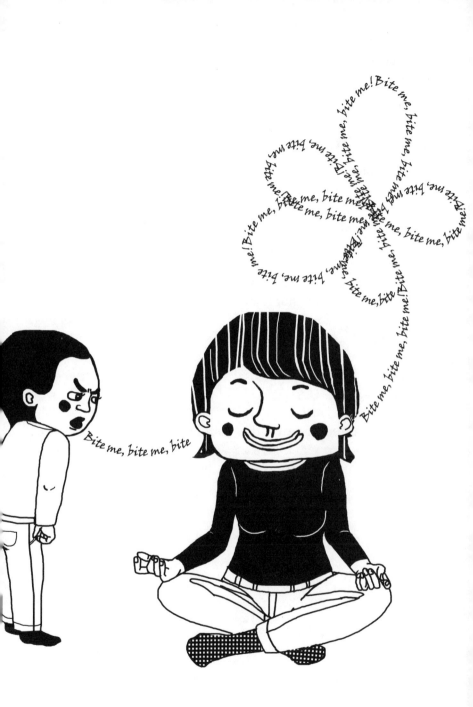

It's good but it can be hard when it's bedtime and he tells me that he isn't going to say good night to me; when he pulls the blanket over his head and pretends that I don't exist. In that case I'll try to make up with him because I don't like going to bed without making peace.

New thoughts

My first thought when I tried this was: Can it be that simple? Then I started wondering why I hadn't thought about it myself. I'm someone who tries every possible solution in order to find a model that would work for us in our conflicts.

Why is it so hard to find the right solution?

It might have been because of the fact that using silence is so foreign to me, because I think that I would normally talk myself out of difficult situations. Perhaps communication doesn't solve everything, and just letting things be is a new way of thinking for me that I am considering.

I've gotten better at asking others for help and tips; not all things work for me, but sometimes I think of something that might help.

I have also become less afraid of making mistakes when trying out new things—no one is going to die if I don't get it right, hopefully we'll have something to laugh at.

What I have also learned is that I am much less anxious now when it comes to my next child. Perhaps Will's and my methods will work, perhaps not, but it doesn't matter. We have to find our own solutions when the time comes.

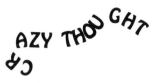
CRAZY THOUGHT

Extra everything!

In our family we are in a place where negativity dominates positivity. We use punishments instead of rewards. We yell and shout, rather than laugh. We are locked in and have no keys!

Kristin with Peter, 11 months, Sara, age 7, and Will, age 11.
I started to realize that our home was full of noise, nagging, and fighting. I talked to friends about it who had also experienced similar issues in their homes. I received some good advice, but it hasn't worked for my family. I've bought instructional parenting books containing ideas and "smart" methods from experts. I've tried a lot of things in my mission to become a happier and better parent, but most of the time I haven't had the energy to follow through and have only half-heartedly tried out some of the methods.

I personally feel that I have a lack of time and energy. I'm currently on maternity leave, but I previously worked a full-time job, and I remember often thinking that you really need three adults in order to run a family. It would be a big help with regard to time and money. It would actually be quite unconventional—three adults living together. Yes, there were two of us, but we had to do the work of three. Besides us two adults, we had a prepubescent six-year-old (is that possible at age six?) and a super-pubescent ten-year-old (is that possible at age ten?) to take care of. We had routines that somewhat worked, but life felt like something that we had to deal with and just get done, rather than something to enjoy and appreciate. Working as much as I did made me unhappy, and I couldn't find anything amusing in working all day, coming home at six o'clock, cooking, and then waiting for my children to go to bed.

My discontent over the situation affected my whole family's mood. The children could see what I was feeling and they seemed to compete at who could test my limits the most. I managed to deal with my children in a decent way three days out of seven, but the fuse blew too quickly on other days. One day we became a family of five; it was a lot of fun but we didn't plan it (okay, so I might have realized it a little earlier than on the day that it was an actual fact). Our frail routines fell apart, and I had even less patience, I was even more tired and couldn't deny the irritation anymore and did everything wrong with my two older children.

Whether it's good or bad behavior, it's easy to fall into routines that become more and more rigid, implanted, and hard to get out of. We continued this way until I had a revelation one day; it was either a spur-of-the-moment inspiration or a sudden what-the-heck. The children came home from daycare and almost immediately began to whine about what they were going to eat for dinner, that they were going to take showers after eating, that they had homework that had to be done, that they couldn't find their clothes that I (!) had lost . . . yada, yada . . . I sometimes enter a state where I look at myself from the outside. I heard what the children said and I heard how they used words as they whined. I had rolled up the fuse wire and hid it in my hair, so that no one could access it and detonate me. I suddenly started thinking of *The Sound of Music* and the perfect, singing von Trapp family.

I felt so happy at that moment and laughing at the misery wasn't hard at all. The angrier the children became, the more I laughed. Not from malice, but from joy. I turned every single negative thing that they said into something positive. It didn't matter how much they tried, it just didn't upset me. I don't really know what happened and how I succeeded, but it was effortless. I was truly happy and it was so incredibly fun and refreshing seeing the children's reactions to my behavior. They didn't understand at first, but pretty soon they looked at me with confusion. They must have thought that I had had a nervous breakdown (which perhaps I did, but we don't need to speculate on that). My ten-year-old, who is usually really provocative, finally let go and put on a happy face.

He almost seemed proud of his mother who had dealt with the hard situation. My six-year-old, who has a temper like no other, also surrendered and started to laugh. Try being angry when someone constantly laughs, praises you, and feels positive. When my husband came home in the evening, he thought he was in the wrong house and had ended up at our neighbor's (although I don't know if they have a lot of fun there . . .). We were very wacky and really happy. It was as if we were all so incredibly relieved that we had gotten out of something that we all felt was discouraging and sad.

Then what happened?

I would be lying if I said that we were just like the von Trapp family from that day on. None of us could be bothered running around being overly excited and positive all the time, and it's not something that I strive for either; that would be awful! There are many days when I can't stand things, but overall, daily life has become a little merrier and my *Sound of Music* trick works every time. The kids don't always follow, but I feel more satisfied when I don't have to get angry.

When it's time for me to go back to work, I will work part-time. Working a lot isn't worth it for me. I don't have enough energy and I don't want to be there as much, especially if I hiss like a wild cat when I am with my family. I'm glad that we make enough money that I can choose to work less. Material things are of less importance to me if I can keep my good mood most of the time.

New thoughts

Thinking of *The Sound of Music* is fun! I understand Julie Andrews—but not every day. It's interesting to change your own behavior and see how others react. Doing the opposite and choosing to lighten the mood suits my temperament and me. I can avoid more difficult situations that way.

Boys' night

My three-year-old son's whining about me not doing things "like Mom" is about to drive me insane. Okay, Mom is great, but I'm not that bad either.

Patrick with Henry, age 3.

After the first few years of maternity leave and working part-time, it was my wife Sandra's turn to start working more. I had a flexible job and was sometimes able to work from home. We didn't think there were going to be any problems. The only thing was, our son Henry was a mommy's little boy. Especially when he was hungry or tired and Mom's way of doing things was the only way.

I've always had a good relationship with Henry. I was home a lot during his first year and it created a strong bond between us. But some-how—and I would sometimes feel a little bitter about it—he was still mommy's boy. In retrospect, I realize that it actually had more to do with the period of his life than with how I was as a father. But when the fuss and whining started and only Mom could comfort him, I felt irritated. In addition, to be really honest, our son proved to be a bit of a know-it-all. He's someone who likes to point out that I put the clothes on the wrong shelf in the closet, that I use the "wrong" kind of soap, and that my pasta sauce certainly doesn't taste like Mom's. One time, Sandra was going to a conference and wouldn't be home for the night. Henry had cried all week that he didn't want her to go. I certainly reali-zed that it upset her, so I did my best to show her that we would be fine. I was convinced that we would be able to manage. The only question was, how much negative energy could I take?

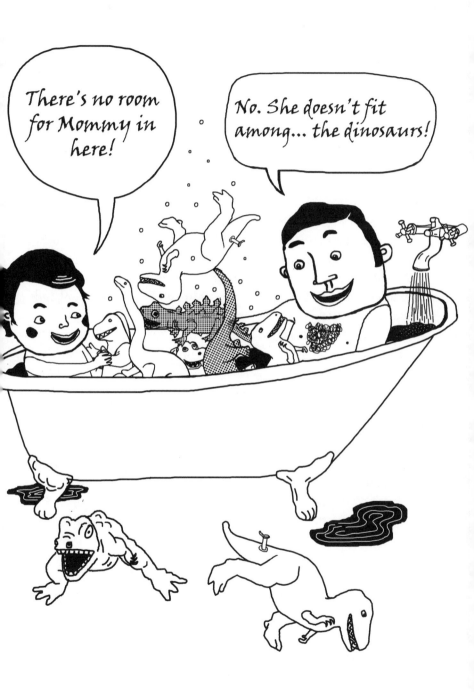

Sandra left early in the morning with a suitcase in her hand. Henry most likely didn't understand that this was the big day, so the departure went relatively smooth. But as the day went on and it was me that had to pick him up from kindergarten this time, he started to become uneasy as he realized that Mom wasn't going to be with us tonight. And sure enough, the crying started at the grocery store. I picked the wrong kind of milk, and he yelled—in an unnecessarily high-pitched voice—that he wanted the green milk and not the red one. Mom always bought that one.

I was standing in the store and I felt how a long and stressful day in combination with a whiny frigging kid (yes, this is what I was thinking in this moment) made my head pound from fatigue. I would never be able to measure up to Sandra's standard, no matter what I did. So how the hell would we solve this? Part of me wanted to take the kid under my arm and just get out of there, another part of me wanted to make another attempt, to talk calmly, comfort him, and be a really cool and kind dad. Take a deep breath and try again.

While I was standing there being indecisive, my gaze fell on a pack of mini-meringues. Why, I don't know—we hardly ever eat meringues at home, Sandra doesn't like them at all, and although I have a sweet tooth, I am not particularly fond of them. But all kids must like meringues, I thought. And I suddenly realized: we were getting meringues!

Henry looked at me wide-eyed as I dropped the bag in the cart. I noted with a sense of satisfaction that he forgot to mention "Mom never buys meringues." I knew exactly what we were going to do for our father-and-son evening.

I quickly threw jam and whipping cream into the basket and explained to Henry that we were going to have a real "boys' night," since Mom wasn't going to be there. And didn't Mom hate pancakes? Yes, Henry nodded, it was true indeed. The corners of his mouth even started to rise, as he realized the possibilities that suddenly appeared: a world that was contrary to what Mom would choose, a world where guys decided the rules and what they wanted to do.

The rest of the shopping went smoothly, and the only difference was that Henry and I chose food together that we normally wouldn't eat at home. The stress and anxiety was long gone and I actually really enjoyed it. Maybe I should have felt guilty that we deliberately bought a bunch of unhealthy things and maybe I should have been ashamed of these cheap bribes. But at the same time, I didn't intend to make a habit out of it. And it actually wasn't any worse than any adult's festive feast on a regular Saturday night.

We opened the bag of meringues on the way home already—because we needed food for the journey. The sugar kick helped us both keep our spirits up before the pancakes were done. After dinner, Henry bathed and he was allowed to have all his dinosaurs and plastic toys in the bathtub with him. However, I explained in a careful way, that our way wasn't better than Mom's way, just different. But I still felt a ridiculous amount of satisfaction as we looked at my car magazines and voted on which model was the hottest.

We both giggled at our decision, which we made before reading a story. We ate white bread with jam for breakfast the next morning. We envisioned how Sandra would roll her eyes because it was such an unhealthy start to the day. What did that entail? This father-and-son thing meant that we had an agreement; we wouldn't tell her any of the details. It would be our secret.

Then what happened?

Henry thought our secret pact was exciting. He also realized in a very logical way that Dad's way of doing things wasn't necessarily wrong or bad. Sandra came home and she obviously didn't ask anything about how we had been living while she was away, even though there were small traces here and there. She was mostly relieved that we had done well without her. As a result of this, it was easier for her to travel for work from then on, and Henry wasn't much of a mommy's boy at all anymore. We had "boys' nights" more frequently and they were different each time. They were all based on what we wanted to do and we did them mostly to spend time together rather than for the goodies.

New thoughts

I'm not bad at all, I'm really good! And I'm sure our son thought so, too. But in a new situation, it's easy to fall into the habit of thinking that everything should follow some rulebook. I realized I don't have to care about it or I can write my own. When I am clear about what I want and how I want it, it becomes the truth—my truth.

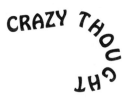

Opposite day

In kindergarten, we talk a lot about what's right and wrong with the children. They are very aware of what's right and wrong, which has its pros, as well as its cons. One advantage is that they learn what to do and how to be in order to function in the society they are a part of. A disadvantage is that they, in their eagerness to do and act right, forget to think for themselves.

Magda, a preschool teacher.
I work as a preschool teacher where we work hard to strengthen the children's self-esteem and confidence. As part of this we want to show the kids that it's okay to do "wrong" things sometimes and that these are often the times that we learn something new. We also want to show that it might be a conscious choice to actually do "wrong." It can be fun doing "wrong," although the words "opposite" or "wacky" might in this case sound better.

We usually have our Opposite Day in November and the last time it looked like this: Wearing pajamas and bathrobes, the staff welcomed the kids in the morning, greeting everyone with a "Bye!" The children were also wearing pajamas. It feels important and gratifying to show that we don't need to be perfectly dressed. Many parents have troubles getting them dressed in the mornings and I think that many children actually enjoy arriving in their pajamas. It does happen that a child becomes a little hesitant and we obviously don't force anyone to take part. Some children need time to figure out what's going on, but then usually choose to join in.

Once everyone has arrived, we snack on sandwiches made to look like pigs, and drink hot chocolate through a straw. Because chairs and tables are upside down, we sit on the table, but on the underside. After snacking, we walk to the store, where "someone" has decorated a Christmas tree and the kids get ice cream and we read stories.

At our preschool, we have the Thursday Box. The idea is that everyone brings something with them from home, only on Thursdays, and puts it in a large box. Then all the children get to show their item and talk about it. We do this because the kids enjoy bringing something with them from home and it's good practice telling a story to their friends. The kids love the Thursday Box and it's an activity they always keep track of. Our last Opposite Day fell on a Tuesday, which meant that we organized a Tuesday Box for the children, and this time we had placed it in the staff room. We adults had put things in the Tuesday Box that we had brought with us. We ignored the one item rule. One of us had chosen to bring loads of things and we ended up with a really crazy and random collection, which the kids thought was hilarious. We ended the activity by singing "Happy Birthday"—even though it wasn't anyone's birthday.

This day consisted of a lot of planned activities and the little time that's left for the children to play was usually the same as any other day. The children played their "usual" games and we hung paintings, lamps, and artwork upside down on the walls. Lunch consisted of Happy Meals, which we ate on the floor in the hallway. At 1:30 PM we moved into the drawing room where we ate breakfast consisting of cucumbers and shredded carrots under an upside-down couch. After a full day indoors, obviously, as we're usually outdoors most of the time, we ended the day with a "Good Morning" as the children left.

Then what happened?

We've celebrated Opposite Day for six or seven years now and we will continue to do so. Several elements have been repeated, but we usually add something new every year. Next time we'll probably try some of our usual games, but we'll change the rules.

We always have fun when we are planning our Opposite Day and we're very cheerful, excited, and energized when we do. We also appreciate all the positive feedback we receive from both children and parents. There is nothing but joy associated with this tradition.

New thoughts

The reasons for Opposite Day are extremely clear; they're even outlined in the curriculum. It's fun to play with the conventions of everyday life—if only for one day. Children love when things get crazy and they are incredibly quick to follow. They get really excited when we let go of our roles and it brings us closer to each other. This is our thing; we talk a lot about it and reminisce. It feels good to do things that are a bit different and that we can look back on.

Stop the nagging

Nagging and cajoling don't work at all anymore. I start to grow tired of my own voice because it's the only thing I hear. I see how my family closes an invisible curtain as soon as I get started. I notice that the more words I use, the more annoying I become.

Peter with Lauren, age 2, and Ellen, age 6.
When I met Lina, I thought that her untidiness was quite charming; it was part of her style. It was a little bohemian in a cool way and very much Lina. I'm not like her, I'm much more conventional; I want things to be neat and organized around me. I was raised with the motto "each thing has its place," and somehow it's ingrained in me.

The first time I saw Lina's apartment I got a shock; it looked like nothing was in the right place. It was all disorderly and not organized. I should have realized the problem then and there and made a run for it, but I was in love already. It didn't take many months before we were living together and Lina quickly became pregnant with Ellen. The clutter and, in my opinion, chaos that surrounded Lina bothered me from the beginning. How hard could it be to stay somewhat orderly?

Her keys always went missing, as well as her wallet, which we spent a long time looking for. We canceled her debit card and later found the wallet in the refrigerator. We talked about our roles at home and who should clean up after whom and which of us should decide how orderly the house should be.

The only thing we ever argued about was cleaning. Then Ellen arrived and we all know what it's like having a baby—I lowered my demands

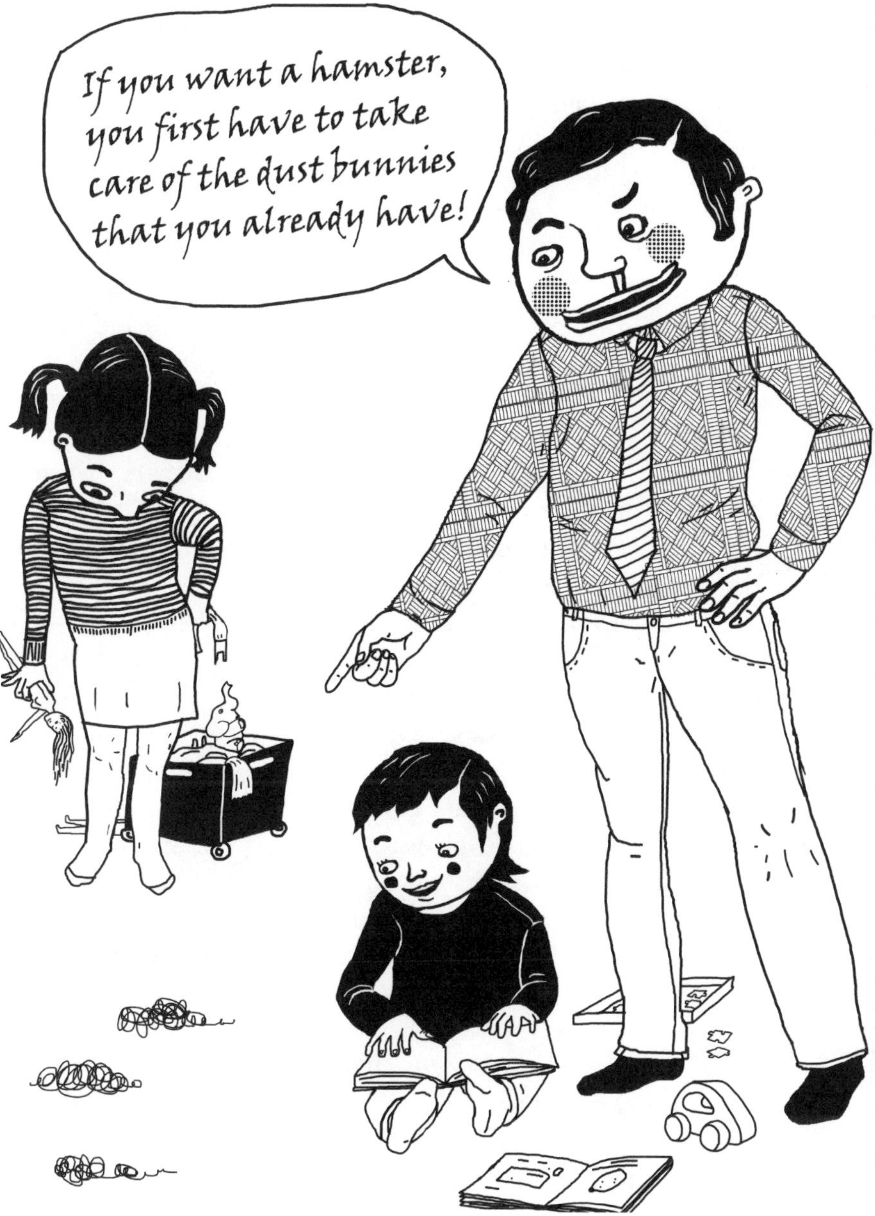
If you want a hamster, you first have to take care of the dust bunnies that you already have!

a lot and Lina did her best to try to maintain a certain standard, like cleaning the bathroom well enough to be able to move around in it. It went pretty well, at least as long as one of us was on parental leave, but when the time had come for kindergarten and work, our house started to decay. I picked things up after Lina, Ellen, and myself. I initiated the Friday cleaning and weekly vacuuming, I had to constantly nag about towels, piles of clothes, empty toilet rolls, and dirty dishes that were all over the place.

I felt like a real whiner who only ever talked of cleaning. What scared me was that I saw the same tendencies in Ellen that I did in Lina, even though she was so young, it was an unconscious messiness and I don't know if she was imitating her mother, or if it was genetic. The only time that we were all engaged in cleaning was when we were expecting strangers; that's when our home looked decent. If Lina's family or my parents visited, we all of a sudden had to clean to make sure that they wouldn't realize that Lina hadn't changed.

But in the end, I got tired of being the inspector general at home so I tried to quit, which didn't work, since my girls carelessly continued living their filthy lives. Getting angry didn't work either, because everyone got upset, and Lina and Ellen promised that they would do better to make me happy again.

At work, there was an older janitor who found a way to make us all remember to clean up our papers, cups, and other garbage. He never nagged us, he never got angry, but he teased us about our cups and candy wrappers in a relentlessly amiable way. By kindly asking if something was ours and asking where he should put it, or should he bring it to the kitchen, he soon created an atmosphere where you double-checked your space to make sure it was clean. He did this in such a kind way that you immediately felt remorse about your own carelessness. You would habitually double-check your desk before leaving, to ensure that there wasn't a coffee cup or any other garbage that he could find.

I decided that I would try the tactic at home, to see if it would succeed. I did it in small doses and didn't tease them about every single thing, but when there were towels in the living room I would pick them up and ask Lina if she had put them on the couch and kindly ask where she wanted them. I did the same thing with Ellen when her things were scattered around the house.

There was a noticeable difference. Lina felt bad and started teasing me because she could pick up after herself, I shouldn't have to. I noticed that both of them started picking things up after themselves more, because I was always friendly and didn't guilt-trip them, but I thought it was quite nice and really enjoyable, since I tried to be pleasant and never accused anyone of anything, which made it easier for me to keep my calm.

Then what happened?

We still have our battles about cleaning and organization at home and probably always will. While other people argue about money or work or leisure, we argue about cleaning. We have two girls now and I hope that Lauren will be more similar to me when it comes to cleaning. Then there could be two inspector generals at home.

New thoughts

It was nice taking on a new role, not having to nag in an unpleasant way but in a nicer way and a completely different manner.

Whose threshold when it comes to messiness will prevail in our family? I'm the only one who has a problem with cleaning; the rest of the family members don't care about the mess. The only thing I can do is ask that they help me with my problem and do it in the most pleasant way that I can.

Everyday life has a silver lining

The majority of our time consists of everyday life. Depending on how you interpret the phrase, and what stage of life a person is in, it may have several different meanings. For a parent of young children, every day looks the same. I find it tedious and dull, not just because it's ordinary, but perhaps more due to the fact that it's so terribly repetitive (and perhaps that's exactly what I associate with everyday life—the repetitiveness). A lot of people choose to "go with it" but I don't want to. I don't want to go through life and not enjoy it, even if it is for a shorter period of time.

Diana with Delia, age 5, and Clara, age 7.
I had tons of ideas about what I would do with my children when becoming a mother. After I actually became a mother, I can safely say that I have slaughtered an entire herd of sacred cows. I've always been pretty calm in my parenting, although I was obviously uncertain and worried when our first child arrived. What really struck me, and what I never previously thought about, was how little variation there is in life when having young children, which is paradoxical, as you constantly face new situations that need to be dealt with. A lot of the times I haven't had the

time to think, and I've just had to go with it. A parent's life is mostly spent at home, with very little input from the outside world.

Before we had kids, my husband and I traveled a lot. We went on adventures, both big and small ones. We always valued being able to be spontaneous and playful. When we had kids, it was as if all the spontaneity and playfulness disappeared. We don't really miss the big adventures. We really wanted to have children and we felt that we made the right choice from the beginning through today and for all time. It's just that the everyday life was about to destroy us. We're two creative beings—or at least we used to be! Can that just go away?

Being creative when you're tired is extremely difficult. That's exactly what happened. We had two children within a couple of years and how much sleep did we get during that period? During my maternity leave, I slept very little, took care of our first child and then the second during the day while my husband was at work. It went well for a long period of time, since I didn't have the time or the energy to reflect on it. Once we got past our second child's baby period, I started feeling and thinking that everything was very gray and regimented. It felt like Wednesday arrived and then it was Wednesday again and again. I think that both of us felt like this, but I had a hard time putting my finger on what it was.

Luckily, my husband came to the realization and decided to do something about it. He came up with ideas and pushed me by arranging what we needed. We put the kids in their strollers and walked down to the ferry boats, got on one that looked fun, and had a fun day. At times we would bring lunch with us but most of the times we didn't bother preparing anything and grabbed something along the way. We would sometimes take a bus one way and walk back home. We ate breakfast at a hotel. We put our indoor cat in a cage and went to the woods to see if she liked it. We ate a fancy dinner and drank wine on a Tuesday. I chose an outfit for the day from the closet while blindfolded. It can be incredibly empowering putting something on other than your ordinary jeans! We visited museums frequently. We rode the entire subway line, because our kids slept so well on the train. We brought books that we read and we would occasionally drift off. A couple of times we opened a map, closed our eyes, pointed on the map, and went there by chance.

The list of the small and exhilarating activities that we did was very long. There really weren't any extraordinary activities, as we didn't have the time, money, or energy. It was just a lot of fun, doing something that stood out from the other things we spent so much time on.

Then what happened?

We have continued to put a silver lining on our everyday lives. When the children were young and I was in the same old rut, my husband was responsible for the creative parts. I have more energy now and can be eager at times when my husband is caught up in everyday life. As the children have grown up, they have become involved in coming up with things to do. They are usually very good at finding small, fun, and peaceful things to do. They also ensure that we actually do the activities. When we start to grow lazy, they push us and make things happen. When the four of us help each other with everyday life in various ways, we become very close. It's great that we can take turns. We also create a lot of fun memories. It's obviously easier to remember that Monday when we walked backwards while shopping than a Wednesday when we bought butter, cheese, and milk after daycare.

New thoughts

Life still consists of the everyday parts, but you can liven things up. Doing something out of the ordinary gives me the energy to pay attention and when I do, I am left with new impressions. When I'm affected, it makes me creative and when I get creative, it's easier for me to pay attention to things and do something out of the ordinary. It's all connected and I can start anywhere I want!

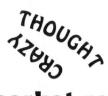

The supermarket race

The day when our family goes to buy in bulk at the supermarket is approaching. We know how it will turn out—whining children who really don't want to be there and two tired parents who would be overjoyed to do something else. The children are too young to be home alone or think that the store is not a horrible place. What a waste having such a boring time! What to do with this dull chore?

Anna and Nick with Wesley, age 5, and Herman, age 9.

There are indeed many musts in life and things that we are obligated to do that we often think are mundane. Our grocery shopping is one of those musts and is, therefore, boring. Our family doesn't deal with boredom very well. We simply eliminate some obligations, but it's hard to ignore the shopping. We've tried splitting up so that one person does the shopping, while the other is home with the kids, but . . . it's tedious. We have tried shopping a little at a time on our way home from work, but . . . it's tedious. For a while, we did the grocery shopping online . . . it was tedious, too.

We realized that we wanted to shop once a week and we wanted to do it together. The fact that it was tedious and we got very tired and grumpy remained. It also felt wrong spending a whole evening once a week on it. That's when we came up with the brilliant idea of "the supermarket race."

"The supermarket race" goes as follows: At home, we write a long list of everything that we are going to purchase. When we get to the store,

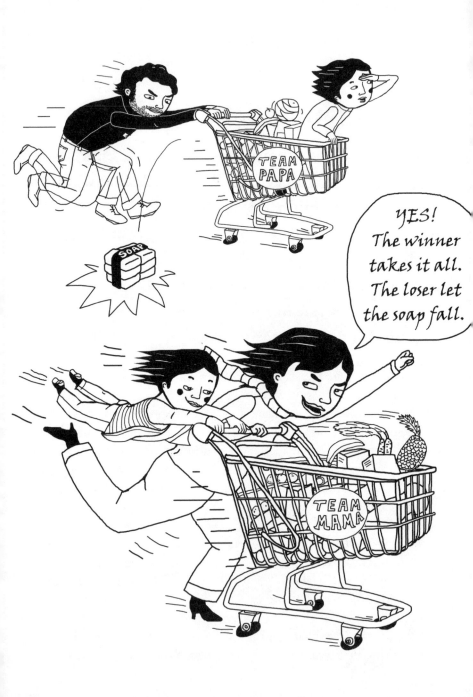

we split up into two teams, tear up the shopping list, and run for it! The rules are simple: The first team to get through the cash register wins!

The first time we tried it, we suggested our idea about the competition to the children a few days before. They were really excited about it. We were also excited and, competitive people that we are, both of us wanted to win.

After that, all we had to do was go around the store with the kids running beside us or standing on the edge of the cart. Pretty soon we figured out that the best strategy was to leave the cart and treat it as a base, and then run off and go find stuff and come back with the goods. It was a lot of fun running into each other down the aisles and peeking at how much the other team had in their cart.

You also had to make sure to carefully look through your list so you didn't forget anything and risk being disqualified. Then when you put everything on the conveyor belt at the cash register you hoped there wasn't a trainee sitting behind that particular cash register or that the receipt roll was running low. The first time we tried it out, we had decided to meet at the cash register by the exit, where they sell lottery tickets and tobacco. We ended up at the cash register line nearly at the same time but we finished about five minutes apart.

The kids enjoyed the actual shopping, but our son who was on the losing team, was sort of grumpy when he realized that he had just lost. When we suggested our contest idea, the boys obviously wondered what the prize was for the winners. We had decided that pride was the only prize, and that we did this because we wanted to play and have fun, rather than compete and win. But they're our kids and like I said, we're competitive people. It wasn't that bad, however, and we could cheer them up with ice cream. It felt like a fair reward, as we managed to do our weekly shopping in less than half an hour.

Then what happened?

We have continued doing our supermarket races, but we have modified the idea a little. After the first time we realized that our younger son had a bigger challenge than his big brother and we therefore introduced a handicap system. The younger son's team would have a slightly shorter list of groceries. We started letting the children name their team, which they really enjoyed. We also noticed that it takes longer shopping for fruits and vegetables, because they have to be packed in bags. We always try to put a bit of thought into the list, to ensure that it's fair.

When we told others about our "supermarket race," we received a lot of positive feedback. Several of our friends have embraced the idea and modified it to suit their families depending on how old the children are. If you have younger children, one version is to cut out pictures of food and let the kids search for the item in the picture. If you have teenagers, they can compete against their parents. The other day we heard about a family with teenagers who tried it out and they managed to do their Easter shopping in fifteen minutes! If you have very young children, the adults can actually compete against each other, because what little kid wouldn't enjoy Mom and Dad going crazy and racing around with them in a shopping cart?!

Others have asked us if we find it embarrassing running around the store like crazy people. We have answered that question truthfully; you need to be young at heart to be able to do this—and we are. You have to be comfortable running about in the grocery store among tired and occasionally grumpy people—and we are. We don't care, as long as we're having fun.

New thoughts

A trip to the grocery store doesn't have to take a long time. It takes time packing fruits and vegetables into bags. You may want to tone down the competitive aspect slightly, depending on your children. If the children are at the age when losing is equivalent to disaster, you can possibly modify the "supermarket race" to suit the needs of your children. This is supposed to be fun!

To compete and play while doing boring tasks has been our salvation.

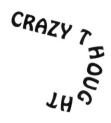

Pursuit racing in the hallway

Our mornings in the hallway are everything but relaxing. This is due to several factors: everyone is in a hurry, and by everyone, I mean seven people, and the hallway is too small. All this chaos leads to conflict, which is, as we know, a bad way to start the day.

Jennifer with Michael, age 2, Vanessa, age 5, Steve, age 9, Axel, age 11, and Leo, age 13.

Before I start telling the actual story, I have to share some of my concerns that existed before we introduced pursuit racing in my family.

The pressure of competing—we encouraged competitiveness in our family, but what we really wanted was for the competition to stop. It became very contrary to what we as parents saw as a solution! Someone is constantly going to be a loser—the whole thing results in the risk that one kid will constantly be behind. It could be remedied by using some sort of handicap system. Despite these concerns, I still believed that pursuit racing would be suitable for us.

To learn about this system, I had to read up a little bit about pursuit racing. I read the following online: "Pursuit racing is where competitors or teams are either chasing after each other or chasing after a lead competitor or team." So far, it pretty much sounded like our family if you replace sports with family life. It continued: "It's the same thing as a team start; the person who reaches the finish line first, wins." Now I began to understand what we have been doing in the hallway over the years—team starts! Furthermore, I read: "The difference is that during pursuit racing, the contestants can begin one after another, usually with a time difference, which is calculated according to their previous results" (like the amount of time spent in the shower and bathroom).

At this point it started getting complicated. I pictured us sharing the hallway with referees in uniform holding stopwatches. Or would I have to act as a judge on a panel? It might be a really nice task compared to arguing with the kids!

At this stage I had already figured out that I couldn't handle the administration of all of this. We'd just have to get rid of the start time, which we had "calculated according to their previous results." We would have to start consecutively with a time difference calculated by their father.

This required some preparation, which was fine considering that I was expecting amazing results. The three oldest children needed to be informed and we would take care of the two younger ones, as they still didn't keep an eye on the time and because they competed to not be in last place.

The first person out was our eleven-year-old who's naturally fast. He started by taking the dog for a walk. While he'd be out, his little brother, who was nine, would come out. He'd take his time—school bag, gym bag, gloves, jacket?! When he started, our teenager's friend came over to pick him up. This was something I hadn't really thought of—another person in the hallway—from the outside. I move him to the side while we waited for our teen to start. He's on his way but he certainly isn't in the starting area. He'd be running around in his underwear, doing his hair, packing his bag, and . . . well, I don't really know what he was doing. I felt sorry for the friend in the hall but he seemed calm standing in his corner with his bangs. Eventually, our teenager was ready to leave. While he walked out the door, a friend of the eleven-year-old's passed through the same door. Another factor I hadn't thought of. He was, as always, in a good mood and instinctively waited in the corner while chit-chatting with the rest of the family. Oh, great!

We were running late, it was taking too long for some members of the family. Our teenager hadn't understood the fun part of the competition at this stage! We took out our young girls' clothes and put them on the floor. When they were about to crawl into their overalls, our dog and eleven-year-old stepped through the door. This is when everything collapsed and went back to normal.

Then what happened?

Parts of the idea of pursuit racing live on. The hallway can at times feel harmonious in the morning. These are brief moments that pass by—they're easily missed. Before trying it out, I thought that we could use the pursuit race in other contexts, such as in the shower and bathroom, but I've had to reconsider—again.

New thoughts

Some things in life are chaotic. I like chaos at times and it's actually one of the reasons why I decided to have a big family. That thought usually helps me cope with my parenting. If the hallway gets too crowded, I can always leave for a little while. I don't have to keep track of everything going on there! Moreover, young children don't understand pursuit racing.

Turn down the volume

When you've gotten used to something, you stop noticing it. I've become oblivious, both when it comes to the color of the wallpaper in the hallway and the noise level of my kids and myself. I can't see that the color is an ugly orange and I can't hear that my children are yelling in the store, because I don't realize it anymore.

Anna with Morris, age 3, Clara, age 4, and Louis, age 6.
Who said that you can't be happy with your big, noisy, rowdy family? Cory and I mixing our genes probably wasn't the best idea for humanity, and perhaps not for our children. I usually say that we're two people with adult attention disorders, who are blessed with three sweet, incredible, yet ridiculously active children.

We are a fun, restless, and noisy family with lots of excess energy. For us, there is no such thing as a quiet time at home.

The fact that the children were born so close to each other has also meant that sometimes there has been more chaos than necessary. When I read a journal I've kept from the time when they were really young, I really don't know how we did it. We had an everlasting struggle of breastfeeding, feeding, nonexistent sleeping, carrying the children, nightly walks, and changing diapers.

Now I can look back at the time in a romantic light, where the children were young, sweet, and happy, but it really was a tough time. I have suppressed a lot and that's probably the way it should be.

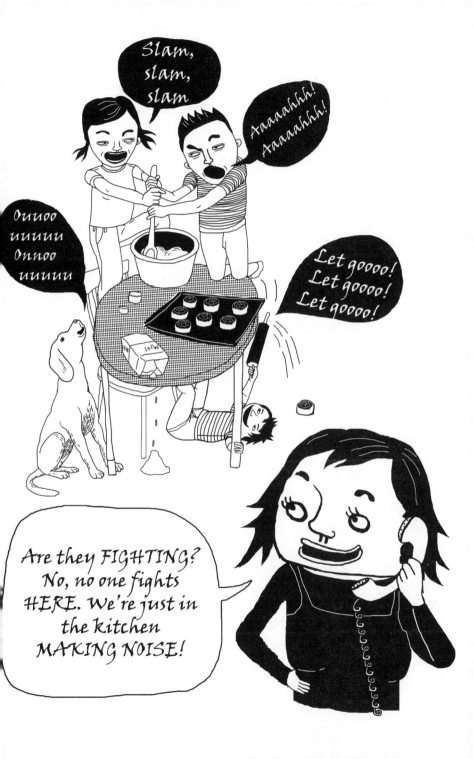

It's constantly a struggle, but these days it's more about the kids questioning what I say and do and trying to juggle kindergarten, work, and home.

Everyday life must go on so they don't get many choices, sometimes no choice at all, but they just do as I say in order for us to get ready and be on time.

I want them to think analytically and be independent, so it's an ongoing battle between us when it comes to wants and needs. We don't always want to go in the same direction, and it's an eternal wait for siblings who haven't gotten dressed or need to go to the bathroom before leaving. Morris has become the best at getting dressed because he got sick of constantly waiting for the other two.

It might sound as if everything is a struggle, but it's really not the case. We do lots of fun and crazy things together. We laugh a lot and play a lot together. With all the energy we carry with us, we end up participating in a lot of chasing games that include running, screaming, and laughing. I want everyone to be happy and cheerful and I have an image that sometimes pops up in my head from the time when Morris was a baby, where I was standing in a bouncy castle, jumping with the two oldest kids, while breastfeeding Morris and kicking a ball for the dog. I know, totally crazy, but that was my life! Sometimes it's still the way it is, but not as crazy.

We and the children are never bored, but we never get any alone time. Louis has just gotten a lock on his bedroom door with the stipulation that he has to open the door if Mom or Dad tells him to, so that he could catch a quiet moment without his siblings. It works well and he really does need his own time.

We try to do things together with one child at a time, so that they get alone time with us. Our alone time as adults occurs at work and every second Friday night when we take turns being away from the family. Otherwise, we would sit on the couch and sleep like so many other families do. When Cory has Friday off, the kids and I usually organize a disco in the living room, which they love but we probably look really silly.

We are probably an unconventional family to many people, just by being ourselves. The contrary thing I usually do is have an argue-free week in order to break free from our rowdy habits, especially at the dinner table. I don't want to scream, I don't want to have fights, but it becomes a way of being. A habit that's hard to break.

We have tried "talking really loud" but it turned out to be complete chaos as the children shouted even louder. We have tried the whisper game and communicating with charades, and that hasn't been too bad. It works the best when the whole family agrees on a week with no yelling or shouting.

During the week of no yelling, neither Cory, the children, nor I get to raise our voice at one other. It's really hard at first, especially for the children, but also for us grown-ups, as it's easy to forget, so we have to remind each other.

I sometimes need to have something in my hand that I can squeeze in order to keep my calm, or Cory and I will "take control" when one of us isn't able to manage. It takes one to two days before the kids start to keep the volume down, calm down, and start lowering their voices.

I am able to say the same thing as I normally would in a loud voice, but because the noise level and my tone of voice are different, they listen to me in a completely different way. I feel educational and interesting to listen to. I would save a lot of energy if things were always like this; being angry takes a lot of energy and doesn't create any respect, since I merely get anger in return.

Then what happened?

We still have weeks when no yelling is allowed, but it's hard to keep it up in our everyday lives. It gets better for a period of time, but then our habits come back, so applying it occasionally works for us. We really need to decide to do it because peace isn't something that comes naturally to us.

I don't believe in having a day of the week with a ban on yelling, since it takes about two days for the kids to start lowering the volume. We have to have occasional training weeks.

New thoughts

We constantly need new ways of thinking and other parents are a great resource for fresh ideas. I often ask others how they handle various situations and then I will pick what seems best. I often try to think in new ways, different is fun. Some things don't work at all in our home, while other things work great once, but no more than that.

Sometimes it's hard to look ahead when living in the present as much as we do, and that may perhaps be one of the reasons why it's difficult to break negative patterns, such as our arguments during dinner. I acknowledge the advantages for the future if I change certain things. But I don't have the energy because in this moment I am here and I can't be anywhere else.

Say YES!

It's so much more fun saying yes than no! But is that a little provocative when we're talking about parenting? We know the importance of restrictions, rules, and routines; no means no and children benefit from consistency and boundaries. I wonder if that's why parents often feel that it's so difficult to take back an accidental "no." We think that the reason that we say "no" more often than "yes" is because as parents, we want to take the safe option. There is a general acceptance of a parent who says "no." As a parent, it's sort of a good thing being able to call the shots—and who doesn't want to call the shots and be looked up to? This entire argument is based on the notion that the opposite would entail being inconsistent, having no rules, and being an inexperienced parent—a nonsense-speaking yes-man. It's nonsense! But what if a "yes" often outweighs a "no"? Do we have the guts to try it out or are we ruining our kids for life?

A brave woman over fifty told us about when her children were young and someone at the Child Health Center told her that breastfeeding more often than every four hours would ruin her children's lives, turning them into spoiled monsters. She was young and she listened, but she felt that both the child and she needed to breastfeed more than every four hours, so she went with what she and the baby felt. When she came to the Child Health Center, they asked how she was doing and she assured them that the breastfeeding was going great and the nurse assumed that doing it every four hours was the solution and that this would produce a healthy child. The courageous woman's children are adults now, and they are well-functioning people without any spoiled monster tendencies. That's the way it worked back then. We can sneer and laugh at the unreasonable rules of breastfeeding at specific times. The theories are so stupid! Imagine what it's going to be like in thirty years, when parents and experts scoff and laugh at the fact that at the beginning of the 2000s, people believed that it was very important for parents to be consistent and have clearly defined rules and procedures. Some people took it as far as putting their children in the corner (which we might already be laughing at)! He who laughs last, laughs best.

The way we look at parenthood and parenting is constantly changing. We have said it before, but whose outlook do we want and who will make the change? We are the greatest experts in the field, and we should, as much as we can, be the ones who make the change and take things forward. In this moment, we are the ones who create tomorrow's history. And if we have to create it in secret, it takes such a long time. Think of all the parents who were told that they could only breastfeed every four hours, and then, in their own homes, completely ignored the recommendations and went with their own feelings and breastfed whenever it suited the baby and themselves. There were probably quite a lot of them. What if they had been open about it, and spoke up about what they were doing and what way they were thinking. Simply protesting against something they knew was wrong. We are well into the 2000s and we do get to think whatever way we want and express it. Progress is a bit quicker these days. We no longer have to hide the fact that we enjoy saying "yes" and that we sometimes say "no" at first, and then all of a sudden change our minds and say "yes," which goes completely against the consistent way of thinking. We can pat ourselves on the back and say with pride: "I love saying 'yes' and I am occasionally an indecisive parent!"

We have thrown out the whole gamut of rules, limits, and routines (which we certainly have praised in other parts of this book), but we know that you're smart and that you'll make your own interpretation of it all. We want to encourage new ways of thinking when it comes to parenting, stimulate new thoughts, and awake the fighting spirit, all in order for you to find your way of being a parent and have the courage to be proud of it. We don't want to preach about what's right and wrong in parenting.

If you are a parent who actually likes certain structures, who feels that it's something that children and parents benefit from—is it then also possible to be a yes-man? Of course it is! Saying "yes" to yourself and your children often makes things much easier, when we know how we want to structure it all. Once you know what your limit is, you can do whatever you want within those limits. You'll know when to say "no" and if you feel uncertain, you can always give yourself some time to think about it (because rapid answers aren't necessary for good parenting). Once our limit is reached, we'll stand there, motionless, while letting our children meet us there. We won't confront, but will just stand firm. We stand firmly on our own two feet, where we've decided we want to be. In order for you to reach your and your children's common ground, you can ask yourself these questions: What does my child need? What are my needs as a parent?

Saying "yes" to yourself and your children sometimes means saying "no" to others. When one mother had her first child, she constantly breastfed for a long period of time. That's what it felt like at least, and it started to become a little frustrating and boring to just sit there with her breasts in the air, so she read a book. An acquaintance came to visit the baby and the new mom described how well it worked breastfeeding and reading simultaneously. The acquaintance responded with: "You can't read while breastfeeding her, because if you don't constantly look at your child, the child will be autistic." It was a comment with the best of intentions that left a trace and made the mother worry for quite a long time. A comment without any evidence, which doesn't help a new parent whatsoever, but mostly makes her feel guilty and worried that she might have harmed her child for life. Therefore, we might need to say "no thanks" to others' ideas in order to be able to say "yes" to our own. It's obviously easier having a set opinion and we may not always have one as new parents, but we are responsible for not allowing ourselves to be told what to do.

Another parent writes on Facebook that her children are rambunctious and disorderly right now and she gets a list of advice and tips. That wasn't what she wanted. She just wanted to air out a little of her frustration. She didn't write: "Help me! I need some advice now! Give it to me, because I don't know how to deal with it!" The comment that she appreciated the most was someone telling her she was a good mother and that her kids were great. That is what she needed in that moment.

Saying "yes" is about affirming yourself and your children. But it's also about affirming the other parent, which is something that can be just as difficult. Are the kids going to turn out worse because we are two different parents? Is one of the parents the expert? What happens to our children if the other parent does things in their own way? One father told us about his first child. His wife had two children from before and was therefore more accustomed to babies, and she interpreted all the signals much faster than he did. "She's hungry!" "I think it's time to change the diaper!" "She's tired!" The father didn't get the opportunity to try to learn the baby's language and interpret her signals because the mother was always one step ahead; not out of malice, but just because she wanted to make it as easy as possible for the whole family. We do it with the best of intentions and love and with a sense of knowing what's best.

Listening to someone is saying "yes" to that particular person. It's amazing being the one who's heard and it's wonderful listening. To be listened to is to grow—I am acknowledged. I become someone by someone else being there, just for me. What I say means something.

Just like us, our children need someone to listen to them more so than someone who solves issues. Continuing to listen without judging and correcting takes skill. Our children have told us many stories as if they were true, but we know are sort of made up and sometimes a pure lie. There is the little boy who one night got to go into the woods with his dad. They sat in silence and looked out for animals. They got to see foxes as well as deer, which was exciting for a four-year-old. When he got home, he really wanted to explain just HOW MUCH of an exciting time he had, and he exaggerated and added some rhinos to the story, so his mom would really comprehend what happened. This particular father kept a straight face and so did the mother: "Well, that's awesome, I hope that I get to see them too when I'm in the woods!" And honestly, when telling a story, does it have to be one hundred percent true? Spicing it up makes it better!

The ability to listen to and follow our kids to have their own thoughts and actions, from the most serious subjects to the silliest games, is about compassion. When we take part in their thoughts and fantasies, we are opening up to new ideas and helping them overcome obstacles that initially may have seemed insurmountable. As parents, we can use our compassion in order to spontaneously be able to put ourselves into situations that are difficult, sad, and scary but also into things that bring joy, laughter, and anticipation. Being able to empathize with the people we meet enriches them, but also ourselves.

As you can see, the yes-saying has many downsides. We are also taking a risk when we start saying "yes" instead of "no," if that's what we are used to saying. We don't know at all what will happen. But if we never try, we'll never know.

Find out when you want and can say YES!

When do you want to say "yes"?

When do you want to say "no"?

What do you need more of in order to say "yes"?

What do you need less of in order to say "yes"?

Workwear

Do you have to wear the same disgusting shirt every day? I'm tired of the never-ending battle deciding whether it is dirty or just stained. As a mother, I want Lenny to be well dressed and I want others to see that he has a lot more clothes than I dress him in.

Charlotte with Lenny, age 4.

When Lenny was three years old, what he wore started to become incredibly important to him.

He'd go completely crazy if the right sweater wasn't clean. He didn't care as much about jeans, socks, and underwear, but his obsession with sweaters was driving me crazy.

He wouldn't wear a particular sweater because it was too ugly or had an irritating tag that chafed his neck, and even though I removed all the tags, something was always wrong. The color was wrong, the pattern was ugly, and this is how it went on. It was the same thing every day. I wanted him to wear various outfits so that it would be obvious that I was a good mother who washed and bought clothes for my son. But to Lenny that was completely irrelevant, so we had a constant power struggle.

According to Lenny, he had about three T-shirts that were good enough and a thick sweater with a Spiderman print that he wanted to wear every day. He loved the Spiderman sweater unconditionally. He wanted to wear it to kindergarten every single day. Stains, dirt, and the fact that he had worn it for three days in a row, those things didn't matter in his world, because that's the one he wanted to wear. At any cost.

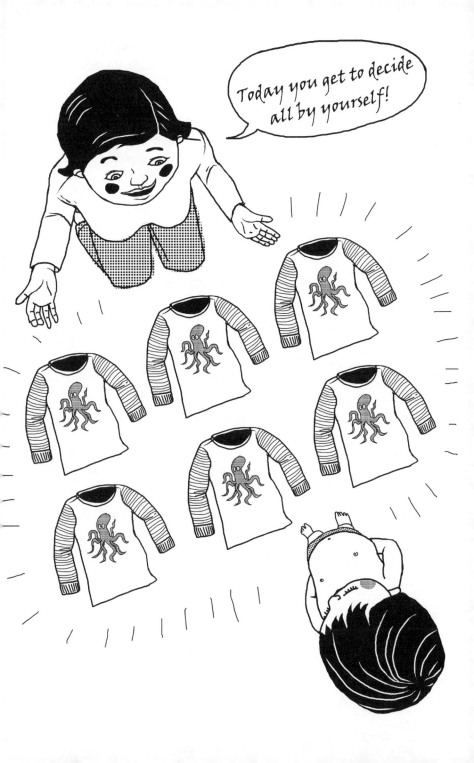

When the sweater was dirty, it was hard for the both of us. There were many evenings when I would be rubbing stains in the bathroom so that it could be used the following day. I knew how important it was to me to like the clothes I wore to work and how hard it was when I didn't feel secure and stylish in my outfit. I noticed the same feelings in Lenny and could actually identify myself with him and his agony, and that's probably why I agreed on doing the never-ending washing.

When Lenny started to grow out of this amazing Spiderman sweater with the faded and peeled-off print, we went shopping twice to buy new shirts. There was plenty to choose from. Lenny was in sweater heaven.

He tried on lots of them, but there was one problem after another with the sweaters. There were tags that chafed him, the wrong fit, a weird color, or it wasn't a hoodie. Because that's what he decided was his new favorite, a hoodie. But then the perfect sweater appeared; I saw it as soon as he put it on. He patted it, put up the hood, moved his head back and forth and sideways to ensure that it wasn't going to irritate him in the back of his neck. But this amazing blue sweater lived up to his standards. He nodded and gave me the thumbs up and I felt so happy; it was a sweater that was good enough! He didn't find any other ones that lived up to his expectations, but he was so happy with the cool new sweater that he had found and already put on.

At that moment I came up with a genius idea, so when we were about to pay, I grabbed two additional identical sweaters. When I was at the register, I had three blue hoodies in the same size; the cashier might have thought it was a little strange.

We had found Lenny's regular sweater; one that he felt stylish and secure in, which meant that there was less work for me, since I didn't have to keep track of whether the sweater was dirty or not, as we had three of them now.

Then what happened?

This thing of buying three identical sweaters has made us both so happy. There is no fuss about clothes, as usually one sweater is clean or at least pretty neat. We've actually done the same with T-shirts. We went to buy some new ones and Lenny came so he could do the neck test and then we bought five identical ones.

What I've realized is that this thing with Lenny's clothes was very much about me, because I always made sure to tell everyone in kindergarten that he did actually have other clothes and that we have many of the same kind, so that they wouldn't think that he only owns one sweater. I know it's ridiculous but I find it hard to resist. I also think that Lenny has gotten better and that he is willing to wear other sweaters. It's still very important to him which shirt he wears, but he considers my suggestions, too.

I think that a lot of it came down to his security and control over things, and his sweater became his security during that period of time.

New thoughts

For whose sake does he need to wear different clothes every day and is there something wrong with feeling safe and stylish wearing the same shirt?

I've been thinking and talking a lot with others about the clothes topic and how important or unimportant it is. Some people really use their clothes as a shield or hide behind a brand; others couldn't care less. Yes, this has inspired me with a lot of philosophical thoughts, but maybe it hasn't done the same to Lenny, who at the moment just thinks that it's important to feel comfortable and be satisfied with his shirt.

The sweater symbolized so much for Lenny; it became his security blanket and protection during a period in his life that was pretty tough. I've also thought about how nice it is to have a work outfit, because you know what to wear. You never have to think about whether it's too dressed up or too casual, because the choice has been made for you. It's quite nice actually.

All Alfonso does is poop!

Children talk about pee and poop—all the time. It might not be the end of the world and is surely a part of it but I'm starting to go crazy! I explain and chastise, but these words just won't go away.

Fred with Jonathan, age 5, and Christopher, age 8.

My sons always talked properly, until I managed to teach Chris a swear-word when he started kindergarten, which I was held accountable for in front of the teacher. Chris quickly learned not to swear and would lecture me every time I swore in front of him. When his little brother Jonathan grew up and was in the age of being fascinated by pee and poo, the boys talked a lot about butts and penises and everything in between, and uttering those words was the most enjoyable thing. Sometimes I felt that they talked too much about pee and poop. I warned them, even though I personally didn't think it was that bad and it was wonderful to see them having fun and laughing. But it can be quite embarrassing when we have visitors or when we go to visit someone. I'm a little ashamed and feel that we have rude kids.

Kids talking about pee and poop when they are in that phase is the funniest thing, everyone knows that. A lot of people don't really mind either, but everyone tries to discourage the children's pee-and-poop talk in front of others. I have explained to my boys that it isn't very nice talking about butts, penises, and farts while sitting down eating and sometimes I get very tired, become angry, and start to yell at them because of it.

One evening, I was reading a bedtime story for them and they giggled when the title had the word "poo" in it. I hadn't thought about it before, but once I started to read I replaced words in the text with all sorts of "funny" words that came to mind. "Dad, can I borrow your fart? Mmmm, but watch out for the dung. But Alfonso just wanted the butt and he didn't touch the dung. Dad continued to pee in the newspaper, while Alfonso pooped and farted." The kids howled with laughter and I couldn't keep a straight face any longer and burst into laughter. The story became completely incomprehensible, but we continued reading the whole book using the funny expressions and the next day they wanted me to read a book in the "poop language" again, which was what they called it.

Then what happened?

I continued to read in the "poop language" every couple of days and it wasn't long before the pee-and-poop talk subsided, and then it pretty much completely disappeared. I was a little worried that they might start talking even more about poop and pee and that they would tell people at school and in kindergarten that dad reads to them in the "poop language." I don't know if they did, but I haven't heard anything about it. I also think that a lot of people try to play down these words too much. It's probably been a year since I read in the "poop language," but new times breed new and exciting words so I think I'll bring the language up to date.

New thoughts

The idea was from the beginning to get the kids to stop using "bad words." How easy is that since I use a lot of them myself? Besides, they're not that bad and certainly not bad enough for us to have fights over it. Keeping abreast of things instead of fighting them is something I use a lot in my parenting. For me it has become a technique that I'm actually quite proud of.

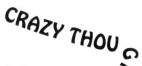

Yes, yes, yes!

Ninety-five percent of my life consists of the word "no." I can't not say "no." I say no before I start thinking about it, and according to my kids, I never say "yes." I personally think that it's incredibly sad when people answer "no" out of habit, without really intending to. I'm sooo boring!

Andrew with Sofia and Ellen, age 6.

I remember that I thought my own parents were incredibly boring and simple-minded because they always said "no." They might not always have said "no," but in my memory, they did. Before I had children, I had an image of myself being a mischievous father who would play a lot with my children and not be very prudish—take each day as it comes. But our first ultrasound, which determined that we would have twins, was enough for me to take the role of the serious, responsible future father of two.

My partner, Lisa, and I were really excited about having two children, but they would be our first children too, so we were a little nervous. I transformed myself into Lisa's knight, who would protect her against all the dangers out there. To some extent, my mission was to protect Lisa, but the more parenting books I read, the more I talked with other parents of twins, and the more Lisa and the babies went for check-ups, the more I felt the weight of the responsibility taking over. I remember that I used to lay awake at night and wonder how I would be able to do everything. Lisa was significantly calmer than me, and in retrospect,

I see that it was probably she who protected me more than vice versa, even though she claims that I was great during the pregnancy.

Sometimes at the maternity clinic our midwife would say, "You'll have to take care of Lisa and ensure that she gets the rest she needs." All I did was take care of Lisa. It would have been so nice if someone could've seen that I also needed to be taken care of a little. Pregnancies are always about mothers! I found it difficult saying what I felt and I did not know how I was supposed to feel, but I would have really needed some "father care" to take care of the anxiety I was feeling.

I started to say "no" far more often than I used to, even during the pregnancy. I turned down everything that prevented me from keeping an eye on Lisa. Sometimes I said "no" on behalf of Lisa too, which made her very angry. "I'm actually still an adult and I can make my own decisions," she would hiss at me. When she told me that, I had no problem understanding that I had crossed the line, but when I did it, I did it because it felt completely right. When the girls were born and they turned out to be healthy and the greatest in the world, both Lisa and I rolled up our sleeves and went with it. For me, it was nice that the babies were in the outside world. It was easier for me when I was able to do something. We were obviously tired, like most new parents are, but we were very excited and it really felt like our large family was a team. I continued reading a lot about parenting, and the idea of the mischievous father who takes each day as it comes, was gone. It may sound like I was really strict, but it wasn't quite like that, and that was probably thanks to Lisa, who didn't let me go down the road of being too methodical.

When the girls were babies, we didn't have to say "no" to them very much, but as soon as they were old enough to walk, Mr. No started reappearing. And that's the way it continued. A part of being a parent is saying "no," but there are limits to how many "nos" a daddy can say. I reached that limit after about five years and don't ask me how many "nos" there were. I started to become really sick of being the one who always had to stop things. My no-saying behavior had also made Lisa become the reliable yes-sayer of the house. Two no-men in the family would've been too much.

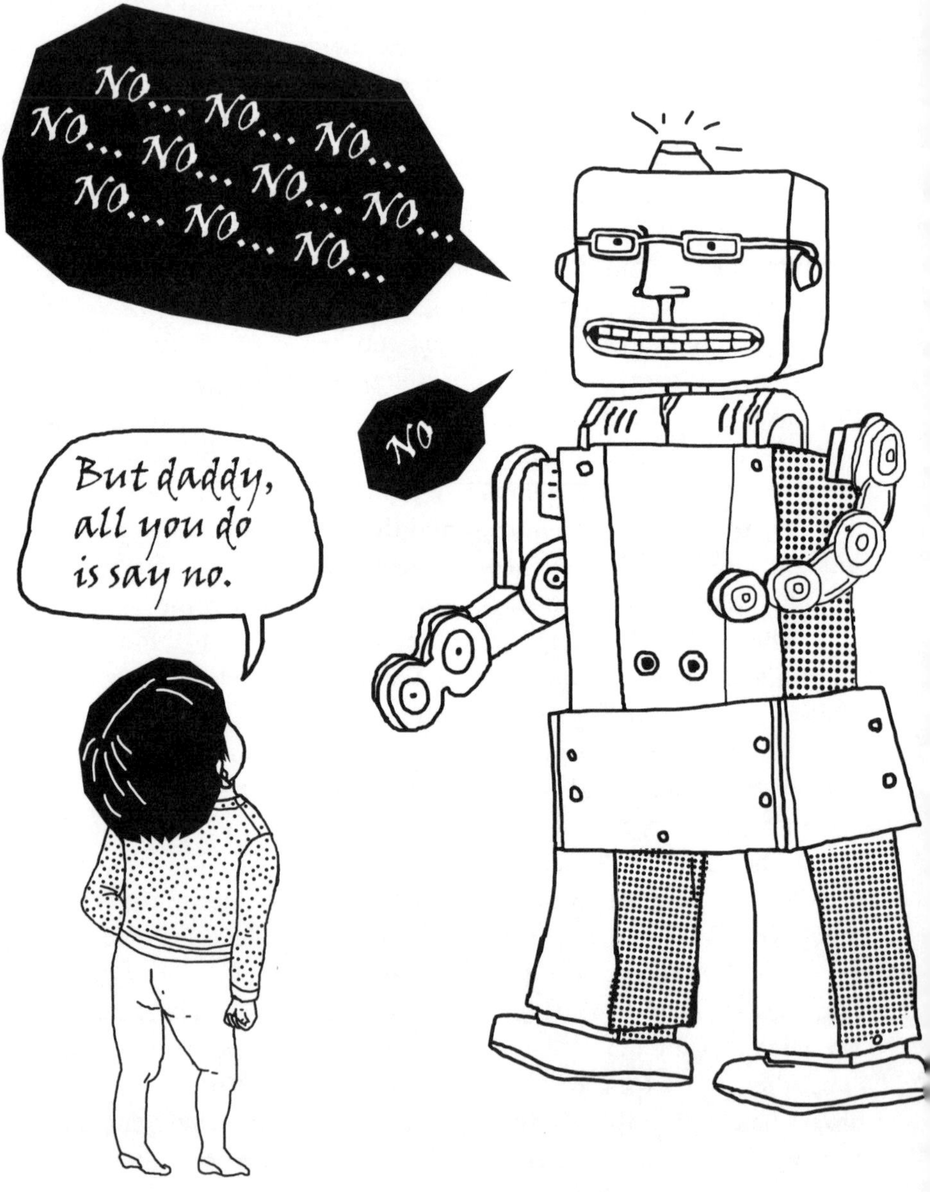
No... No... No... No... No... No... No... No... No... No...
No
But daddy, all you do is say no.

As with all habits and patterns, it's difficult to see how they come about and it's really only now, as I am telling you this, that I realize how this crept up on us. Still, I came to the realization one day when Sofia and Ellen shouted: "You always say no!" I was quick to defend myself: "No, I don't, and what would it be like if no one in this family said no at some point?" If I had teenagers, I probably would've gotten a clever answer to that question. Instead, I got the backs of two very angry six-year-olds. My question left me hanging and in that moment I decided not to be Mr. No anymore.

To start off my new life of yes-saying, I decided to play a game with my family. When was the last time that I played other games than my children's? I decided not to say anything to the others, not even Lisa. From then on, I would only say "no" in exceptional cases, but to start off, I would say "yes" for an entire day. In order not to make the challenge too difficult, I decided to start it during a weekday, as the girls and I would only see each other in the morning and evening. It started out great in the morning, when Ellen asked if she could wear a skirt without tights (this was in the middle of April and it was sunny but only a couple degrees). My obvious response the previous day would have been "no," as it was way too cold outside. But what did it matter—she wasn't going to freeze to death—so I told her "yes." The look on her face! Sophia immediately wanted to wear her thin summer jacket and I said "yes" again. Lisa had already left for work, which was lucky because otherwise I think that she would have stepped in and said "no." I really wanted the girls to know what it felt like when I said "yes."

Sophia asked me at the dinner table that evening if she could leave some food and I said yes, without a doubt—as long as you are full. After dinner they asked me if they could go out, which I would usually say "no" to, as I thought it was good if they stayed inside and got to unwind a bit before they went to bed. "Yeah, go ahead," I said and cleared the dinner table. Lisa now knew that there was something going on and I told her about my experiment. I explained what I came up with and told her that I was tired of being Mr. No. She thought that she was a no-sayer, and we concluded that most parents probably are. We decided to try to think a bit before saying "yes" or "no." Lisa wanted to take part in my game and we decided to try it out for a whole day.

Then what happened?

We still say "no," and we intend to continue to do so. I try to think before answering because I easily say "no" out of habit. We've had yes-saying days a couple of times and it's amazing how much you can actually say "yes" to! We've talked a lot with our friends who are also parents and they agree that there are a lot of "nos." Several of them have tried our game and had success. We also talked a lot about how we as parents often are skilled at talking about what children cannot do rather than what they actually can do. If there were 95 percent "nos" previously and 5 percent "yesses," it's probably 50/50 now, and that makes a huge difference. The children haven't found out about our game, but they tell us that we seem happier. I actually feel happier too, and somehow it's like I can venture out now and be the mischievous father.

New thoughts

Getting rid of certain words in your vocabulary, if only for a day, works great. Saying "yes" is enjoyable! It's good to say "no" when necessary. It's nice sharing the no-saying with your partner. There's a lot to be responsible for as a parent. Even fathers may need looking after when they are expecting.

The worst game

My son is in a crisis, and I comfort and console him. But it isn't enough.

Dan with Mika, age 1, Calle, age 6, and Oscar, age 8.
I think having children is fantastic and it becomes even more enjoyable the older they get. There is something comforting and defenseless about them when they're young and think that Daddy and Mommy can protect them from all evil and possible pain. But they have an awakening when they discover that we parents aren't God and that scary things both can and do happen.

My children's awakening came when they were about five, at which point they were in a complete existential crisis. Oscar had an incredible number of thoughts about us disappearing or dying. I remember the many anxious talks we had, often at bedtime.

"Who is going to take care of me and Calle if you die? What would I do if you were gone one morning?"

What did he mean by "gone"? I wondered.

"That I wake up tomorrow and it's empty and only me here?"

How do you respond to all these questions and concerns? Hypothetical questions, according to me as an adult, but to Oscar they were very serious. I would console him and he would feel better for a bit, but it didn't diminish his fears. Concrete, rational answers might work for an adult, but not for my five-year-old son who was caught between fantasy and reality most of the time. He didn't understand that it wasn't going to happen.

"The star that you can see up there is not going to crash into Earth in your lifetime, even if you think it's getting closer and closer." But there was concern in his heart that traveled down to his stomach, which made his carousel of thoughts spin around. It really was a difficult time for all of us.

During that period, when Oscar was five years old, "the worst game" was invented and the whole concept revolved around going with it and not against it. We were on our way to see some friends who had bought a cottage and because we went after work, it was dark before we arrived. Oscar asked me what would happen if our car broke down in the middle of the dark woods. I could hear the anxiety in his voice. So instead of saying that it couldn't break down, we had half a tank full of gas, and the car was fine, I asked him: What's the worst thing that could happen if the car stopped?

"That you and Mom would go and look for gasoline in the dark," Oscar replied.

"But if we have to, what would be the worst?"

"That you leave me and Calle alone in the car."

"What's the worst thing that could happen then?"

"That it's dark and that you don't come back," said Oscar.

"And that a monster will arrive," added his little brother.

"That you die," said Oscar.

"Because the monster eats you up," said his younger brother.

As we ran down the list of all their fears of this darkness, we tried to solve them all: if the car broke down we'd go together, because no one should have to go on their own. But first we would call our friends and ask them to bring gas or help.

Our boy felt safe because of these concrete solutions, and he was able to share his concerns without being comforted, interrupted, or belittled.

We named this game the "worst game" after this incident.

It would involve anything from someone dying or disappearing to the fear of various things. We engaged the boys to state their worst fears and sometimes we encouraged them even more. It was like having a box of fears and picking up something large and slimy, twisting and turning it, and finding your own solutions and new perspectives. While doing this, the fear shrinks and becomes a little smaller the next time. A fear or anxiety doesn't have to disappear, but you can help diminish its power.

Then what happened?

It's worked well for us, we still play the "worst game" sometimes.

The boys have grown up and we don't need to use it when it comes to the serious questions, but it can still be useful, like when Oscar didn't have the courage to sign up for a team sport, what was the worst that could happen?

My wife and I have also used it when it comes to our adult issues, like when Kate was going to give birth to Mica, we talked about all sorts of nonsense and problems. When I lost my job and pictured the worst scenario, we did the same thing. We looked at it as if it was going to bring a huge crisis that would make us lose our home, I would grow overweight and drink too much, and Kate would leave me, and in the end, we couldn't help but laugh.

We have been told that the "worst game" isn't any good and that it makes us worry more, rather than help, and it was Kate's sister who said that. But for us it has been a way to make our worrisome children feel safe.

When I give words to something that's stuck in my head, it becomes less significant and loses its power. I get to express my concerns and get help with finding solutions.

New thoughts

As parents, we wish that our children wouldn't have to face sorrow, fears, and unpleasant things; that we can protect them against pain, but sooner or later our comfort isn't going to be enough, our cotton bubble might not be what they need in that moment.

My thoughts aren't new and life-changing but they are pretty new to me! When I just listen without solving problems, things usually work out by themselves. Listening rather than solving saves me a lot of time and effort. But because society is very solution-focused, that's usually why parents try to be, too. It's supposed to be quick, we have to find a solution, but there might not be a good solution coming from a parent when it comes to monsters in the dark woods.

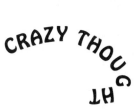

Pretty in a dress

My son loves clothes. He wants to be pretty. Pretty equals a dress, according to him. But according to the social norm, boys should wear pants.

Jack with Olly, age 6, and Sara, age 8.

My wife, Mia, and I have always liked going our own way and we wanted to encourage our children to do the same. Both of us had a lot of opinions on the gender issue and our Olly enabled us to really twist and turn the concept of gender stereotypes. When we had our first child, Sara, we usually dressed her in blue because we thought it was a nice color. I remember how people would look down at her in the stroller and ask, "What's the name of the boy?" And we said, "Her name is Sara." We responded without being the least offended or concerned in any way, and felt proud and happy that someone was looking at our child, our beauty. Despite this, many people reacted by being embarrassed and apologizing for their "mistake." But how would they know what sex our child was? How do you know what sex a baby is when it isn't naked? And does it even matter?

My thoughts on gender most likely arose and deepened when I became a dad and when I, as a man working in a traditionally male-dominated field, construction, chose to go on paternity leave for eighteen months with Sara. When I later chose to work a six-hour day when both Sara and Olly were small, it was such a unique thing that a parenting magazine interviewed me. They portrayed me as a tender macho builder dad with a kid in each arm, standing in the middle of a construction site. It was even better when they found out that I'm a drummer in a rock band. So manly! Interesting!

The older men at my workplace thought it was funny but when I, every day, would leave work to go home two hours before them, I always got the question: "Are you leaving already?" In order to stay sane, I asked one of the older men if he felt that he spent enough time with his children when they were little. He thought about it for a minute and then said, "No, I actually wasn't . . . it's great that you think like that . . ."

I really didn't intend to put my colleague in his place; what parent feels that they spend enough time with their children? I actually wanted to find out what his thoughts were and how he looked at it, disregarding the issue of clichés and stereotypes. Following this, there was rarely anyone who commented on me leaving early.

Olly was about two years old when he started caring about what clothes he wore. Just like many siblings do, he looked up to his sister in many ways. I don't really remember how it all started but Olly probably saw one of Sara's dresses and also wanted one. There were tons of outgrown dresses and it wasn't hard finding one in Olly's size. Olly loved his dresses, and soon, he didn't want to wear anything but nice dresses. Neither Mia nor I initially reflected on the fact that Olly wore a dress. It was just really convenient that he could inherit his big sister's clothes.

We noticed pretty soon that people around us weren't as comfortable with the fact that "Olly, the boy" always ran around in a dress. We had to explain and defend ourselves to many people. Mia's father wondered if "it really was healthy to let the kid wear a dress." Acquaintances would say with a slight smile, but with much seriousness behind the smile: "You never know what could happen if he gets used to wearing a dress." What we considered being nice and positive suddenly turned into something we needed to consider and actively take a stand on.

I especially remember when there was a costume party at Olly and Sara's kindergarten. Olly was just about two years old and he immediately knew that he was going to dress as Barbie. At the kindergarten, the teachers greeted him.

"Hi Olly, what are you dressed up as today?"

"I'm Barbie," said Olly.

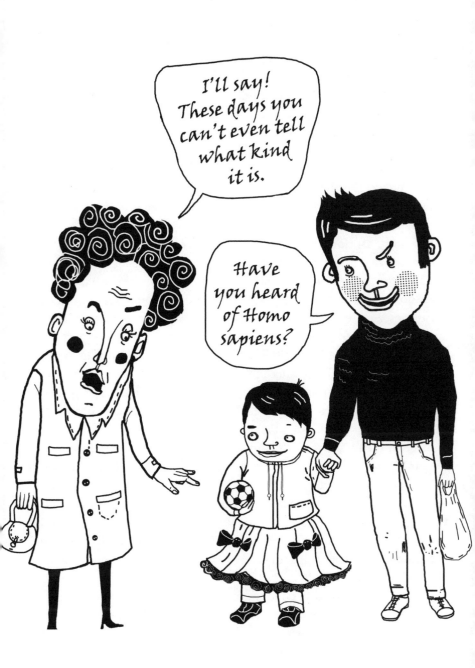

"Oh, you're a baby!" they corrected.

When I went to pick Olly up in the afternoon I was told how the staff the whole day had assumed that he had dressed up as a baby. I explained that he wasn't a baby at all, but Barbie. Everyone now realized why Olly had been in such a bad mood all day and angry about being called a "BABY!" Poor kid, the frustration of it! Being taken for a baby when you're just old enough to understand that you're absolutely not a baby anymore. I don't know if I was right, but I couldn't help but think of what the teacher would have heard if a girl told them she dressed as Barbie. Would they be more inclined to hear her correctly? Like I said, I don't know, but maybe it would have been easier to hear Barbie in that case?

Mia and I sat down and talked about Olly's dresses. We just wanted him to be whatever way he liked. We compared our beliefs to others'. What if he turned out to be gay or a transvestite? We quickly realized that it was nonsense and if it happened to be that one of our children turned out homosexual, would it make a difference in our secure view that our children should be whoever they want to be? No, we'll always respect our children for the people they are! Then the next thought popped up: How will others react to Olly and his choice of clothes? Do we need to protect him from getting hurt and violated? Yes, we might need to sometimes, but not by taking away the dresses. Who would that hurt and offend? Maybe we would accidentally lose the dresses . . .

After all the twisting and turning, we came to the conclusion that as long as Olly wanted to wear a dress, we would support him—wholeheartedly! Making that decision was a relief. It was in line with how we looked at our roles as parents. We didn't have a problem with our son wearing a dress. We were neither for nor against it. A dress is cool and pretty! Let it be! We have to point out that there were a lot of people who thought that Olly's dresses were fun and that we were good parents who supported our children.

Olly continued looking good in his dresses. They were flowery, pink, and ruffled. Once when he was four, he came home from kindergarten and told us about the older boys who told him that boys don't wear girls' clothes. I remember his face and how he, quite confidently, almost felt a little sorry for the older boys who didn't understand the point and the beauty in dresses. There were several of these incidents and it really strengthened our belief that we were doing the right thing.

Then what happened?

Olly is six years old now and looks like most other boys his age. He wears pants and Spiderman shirts. He stopped wearing dresses at the age of five. I don't know what it was that made him stop wearing dresses. Maybe other people's comments, perhaps his insight into how other boys looked? I don't know if he felt grief or if it was something that just came to him naturally. I don't have an opinion about it, either. Mia and I just hung on and supported him in that decision as well. I personally miss the dresses but I comfort myself with the fact that it was fun while it lasted. I look at our family photos with our great kids looking happy in their dresses and flowers in their hair.

New thoughts

It might not be something new but now I strongly believe that my kids should be able to be themselves. As a father, I will continue to support both my son and daughter. There are issues in life more important than clothes, and we can teach our children that lesson through clothes. In our family the dresses will never "accidentally get lost."

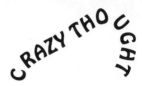

How much fun is it being an adult?

My child doesn't want to go to daycare and I'm trying to understand what it's all about. Has her kindergarten uniform gotten too tight?

Sofie with Mira, age 5.

Mira suddenly realized that she didn't want to attend kindergarten. Nothing had happened, there weren't any mean children or teachers, everyone was nice and she liked it, she just didn't want to go.

I tried having pleasant conversations, serious conversations, angry conversations, but it all had the same effect; according to Mira, kindergarten was completely overrated and she would use her time doing something more worthwhile, like starting school or trying a more mature activity that suited her age more.

I talked to the staff and they didn't understand anything, as she was polite when she was there, took care of the younger children, did things by herself, didn't let anyone put her down, and talked about what she wanted and needed. She was, in other words, the image of the perfect kindergarten child. It was nice to hear that she was peaceful, mature, communicative, and friendly because at home she turned into monster Mira, nagging monster Mira:

"I don't want to go to kindergarten! Kindergarten is boring! Everyone is stupid!"

Every afternoon, every night, not to mention the mornings, we would have the same discussion. We ended up in a vicious circle that started and ended in the same way, with us not getting along and shouting at each other. It really wasn't nice leaving my little girl in kindergarten after our morning fights, so I continued my day with a big lump in my throat and a lot of guilt.

The situation became worse, and I was as grumpy as she was stubborn.

One morning I finally snapped and shouted at her on our way to kindergarten:

"What the hell are you going to do, kid, are you going to start working or something?"

The grumpy troll lit up and nodded, she wanted this very much; there was nothing more she wanted in her life, actually! Why hadn't we thought of this before?

I quickly told her that this was something her father and I had to plan, by tomorrow we would find a job for her. She was satisfied with that, but as soon as we got to kindergarten, she announced that she was quitting, because she had found a job.

"Oh crap," I thought.

I called Joe and prepared him for the fact that our five-year-old daughter would start working to help support the family. He wasn't amused, but understood the importance of finding a job for the kid.

In the afternoon, she said good-bye to the staff and she couldn't say if she was going to return again, but everyone promised her that she would be welcomed back if the job turned out to be boring or if she needed vacation. (We hadn't even found work for her yet.)

We started with a day at my job, in school. Working as a teacher would probably suit Mira. The marvelous functions of the copying machine, which collates and staples papers, were not required. Mira manually collated three papers for the ninth graders and stapled twenty-six booklets with three sheets each, which took a little while, but Mira kept at it. She mumbled to herself, but did not give up, sheet number one, number two, number three, and staple.

My cute helper finished and got lots of praise. After that it was time for a coffee break. During the following two classes, Mira got to dust shelves in the classroom and organized books neatly.

There was a strange stew served for lunch that she didn't like, but she didn't utter a word of complaint; this is what comes with working, there is nasty food but I'll just have to bite the bullet.

In the afternoon, she cleaned the school library, wiped off shelves, organized books neatly, and then she got tired. We went home earlier than usual, as I had a very tired girl with me. She didn't say much in the car or a lot at home either.

Joe was very happy and told Mira that all of his colleagues had organized work for her and that everyone would need help the following day. Mira still didn't say much, because she was tired, so tired.

The next day Mira got to copy papers, lick stamps, clean a shelf, and wash cups in the kitchen . . . then she quit at lunch time. Kindergarten was still like a vacation compared to the slave labor that she had done for two days. Sure, she had been absolutely indispensable and she made money, but she missed her friends.

Then what happened?

It cost us one hundred dollars in wages, but it was money well spent. We haven't heard a bad word about kindergarten after these hard days of work. At times she has said that she is going to go back to work, and we have told her that she's welcome and that there is plenty of work for her at our jobs.

What she said about Joe's job was the funniest: that his colleagues are really boring and didn't laugh at all, and that's precisely what I think, too. But I don't say it out loud.

I also need to pat myself on the back because I've become a lot better at listening and it has reduced a lot of tension at home. Our last fight was last week when she had gotten a haircut and thought that she was ugly. Had this happened six months ago, there would have been a struggle for days in order to get her to kindergarten. Instead, I asked her if she had a solution other than to stay at home and she just shook her head. Then I asked if I could make a suggestion, which meant that I would phone kindergarten to ask if she could wear a hat until she got used to it. Mira approved, even though she would have rather worn a hoodie. I called and we managed to leave without a morning fight.

New thoughts

Things are sometimes a lot easier than what they seem like at first. It's simply a matter of asking Mira of she can solve a problem herself. I often try to find new solutions to problems we can't seem to get out of. I also think that I have become better at making Mira a part of the process, so that she can come up with suggestions because she is a bright person, my daughter.

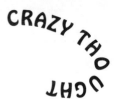

CRAZY THOUGHT

Ice cream before dinner!

Our afternoons are really hard and neither I nor the rest of the family could be bothered with Owen Grumpy Pants. He's tired, hungry, and angry and he tests everyone's patience.

Anne with Owen, age 4, Sally, age 12, and Emanuel, age 14.
When we get home after a long day of work, picking the kids up from kindergarten and grocery shopping, we're always tired.

Our last drops of energy are spent getting home and getting in through the door. There are grocery bags to be unpacked and everything has to continue on. I'm tired and my son is tired, hungry, and angry.

Having to quickly make food with an angry four-year-old while being exhausted yourself isn't an ideal situation. We would fight almost every day. Also, I have older children who have always "helped out" when I cooked in the kitchen and it has worked well, as they were able to chop, stir, and eat vegetables and bread at the same time. This has never worked for their younger brother, who squirms on the floor like a surly ragdoll, falls off the kitchen stool, gets angry, goes on about things, and gets sad, tired, and hungry.

His bad mood continues during dinner where he refuses to eat, teases his siblings, shares his food with the dog, gets upset about small stuff, and is a real pain to everyone. It's been tough on all of us never getting any peace and quiet, and squealing and yelling has become a part of everyday life. The older kids have even asked if they can eat in their room because it's so loud at the table. One ordinary day, it wasn't any

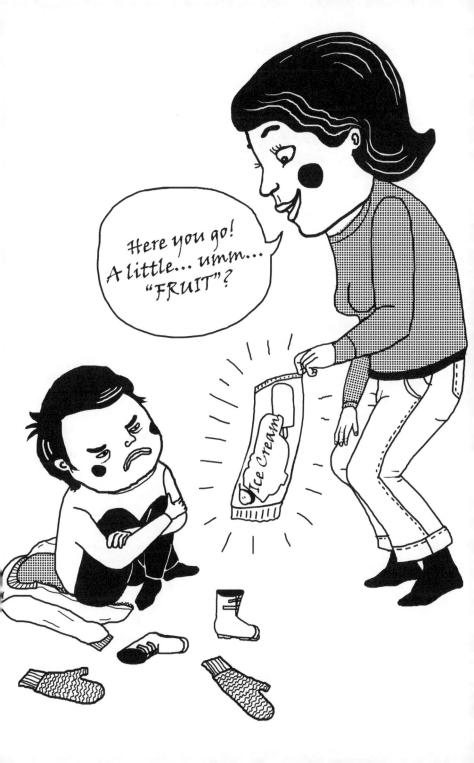

worse than usual, he kept on nagging until his mouth practically dislocated because he wanted ice cream before dinner. I said "no" as usual: "No ice cream before dinner, you can get a popsicle after dinner if you quit nagging."

I don't know what happened to me but I suddenly changed my mind and dug some ice cream out of the freezer and offered him a pear-flavored popsicle. Owen looked at me with big eyes and didn't understand what was going on. Ice cream before dinner? I coaxed in a cheerful voice, not in an angry, "I've-given-up" voice, but in a cheerful and kind voice that urged him. "Go ahead, have ice cream" (because you've worked hard, spending a whole day at kindergarten. I didn't say it, but that's what I meant).

There was silence as he happily sat on the kitchen stool and ate his ice cream. Before he had even finished the last drops from the stick I took out the package again and asked him if he wanted another one. What four-year-old would say no to that? Not mine, anyway.

When he was almost finished with his ice cream, I offered him another one, but he had reached his limit. "I'll have one after dinner if I can fit it," Owen said. He also finished eating his food despite having eaten two ice creams. It wasn't a giant portion but he finished the food on his plate. He was pleasant, which also made me happy. There were no fights at the table and there was no tired kid sliding off the chair. It just worked. A normal pleasant family dinner with your average friendly family.

Then what happened?

Sure, we often fall into the bad habit of whining, but it has become much better on the whole.

An ice cream before dinner keeps Owen's blood sugar at an even level. He becomes friendlier and he even has enough energy to help out at times. The whole family gets to have a better and more comfortable dinner experience, I'm happier, and I have the energy to be nice. So it's positive for the whole family.

An ice cream a day is enough for it to work.

It doesn't happen every day, but I will sometimes even ask if he wants an ice cream when we get home. I think Owen eats better now than he did before. It might not have anything to do with the ice cream, but I can see a change since the crazy idea came to mind. I have experienced positive as well as negative reactions to our family's ice cream consumption. The dentist went bananas, despite his promise that he was brushing his teeth twice per day. Another mother I know tried it out and it worked for her family, too.

Another comment I've gotten is "Why don't you give him fruit instead?"

"Because he doesn't want fruit," I reply. I'm sure it works for someone else, but I can't trick Owen into eating fruit. I've also been thinking a lot about how different we are in terms of our primary needs. Owen turns into a monster when his blood sugar gets too low and I turn into one when I don't get enough sleep. Realizing we have to be more sensitive to each other's needs, I know that it may sound corny, but for me it was an awakening. When a sibling isn't like the others, doesn't respond to the same things that have worked for "everyone" else, how difficult it is for parents to reconsider, think in new ways. But once you do, it can turn out great.

New thoughts

Who says kids don't eat if they have ice cream before dinner? Why have I believed it?

I've also thought a lot about each child's role among his or her siblings, and if this might have been a way for Owen to claim his place among the bunch, wanting to talk and get attention at the same time.

We all want our piece of the cake and my children take their share in different ways.

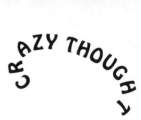
CRAZY THOUGHT

Give your children their own time

For several months my baby has been glued to me. It's been wonderful but now I long to do things by myself sometimes. Every time I do, I feel remorse and thoughts about whether my need for personal time really can be prioritized before my baby's needs for me.

Pernilla with Brandon, 7 months.

Before Brandon was born, I thought a lot about what kind of mother I wanted to be. I wanted to be very present and physically close; I would talk and sing to him. This is pretty much what happened when he arrived into this world. My husband and I carried Brandon all the time and held him skin-to-skin a lot. The only time that he lay by himself during the first weeks was when he was in the baby stroller. At night he was stuck to one of us and when he was awake, we would talk to him and sing a little. When he got a little older, he was more on his own, on a blanket on the floor or sitting in a baby seat. I now discovered the paradox of it all. Would he be okay by himself? What if he felt completely abandoned, unloved, and unseen? What if he would be scarred for life? To compensate for the fact that I wasn't carrying him anymore, I usually tried to have a lot of eye contact with him. I would often find myself sitting in front of him on the floor, talking.

It didn't help that he seemed as satisfied as ever, sucking on his fingers, chewing on a toy or studying a table leg. My guilty conscience arrived like an email in my inbox, when I decided I actually wanted to do some things for myself. I mean, who was more important? When I write about it now, it sounds like I wanted to backpack in Asia or travel through Europe, but that wasn't the case. No, it was things like reading a magazine, taking a shower, reading my emails, or getting completely lost in a phone conversation with a friend. Those little things that reminded me of what it was like thinking of myself—dropping some focus off Brandon.

I was also struggling with myself, as I'm bit allergic to talking about parents having their own time. If you choose to have children, you want to be with them . . . right? What's it really about? Although the issue of parents having their own time has annoyed me, I felt that my previous thoughts were pretty exaggerated and unfair.

In my eagerness to philosophize, I started wondering if Brandon even needed to be left alone sometimes, to get a little peace and quiet. Could it actually be that some alone time would do Brandon good? I completely changed my mind and came to the conclusion that I could with a clear conscience devote myself to personal stuff now and then, in order to satisfy Brandon's needs. I turned it around. It's healthy for Brandon to be by himself sometimes: take in impressions and think through his own thoughts or explore things around him—at his own pace, in his own way. Obviously with me close by, but not necessarily with my face right in front of him.

Then what happened?

It has worked pretty well. I obviously have to remind myself that Brandon's alone time is good for him. It's now a lot easier to tell myself that when my guilty conscience strikes.

Brandon has just started to crawl on his own and giving him his alone time is much harder these days. He's usually doing things that need at least one pair of watchful adult eyes. Sometimes he still gets his own time and this usually happens in his crib, and it's obvious that he likes his own company.

New thoughts

Sometimes you just have to look at things from different angles, in order to accomplish something new. When I think of the fact that I give Brandon a moment to himself, it makes me happy and satisfied.

I think it is wise and healthy for me to be able to turn my thoughts around, so that they favor me. When I feel good, Brandon seems to feel the same way.

The secretly borrowed cat

My kids nearly nagged a hole in my head about getting a pet. I don't want any pets. I don't even like animals. The more I say "no," the more my children nag. I'm not even sure if they would really like having a pet and they may not even know that themselves since they've never had one.

Matt with Daniel, age 5, and Sara, age 7.
I've personally never longed for animals, not even when I was little. Many of my friends really wanted pets and would finally manage to get a bunny or a hamster after pestering their parents. But when they had to face the fact of having to take care of the little animal, it was not as fun as they had expected. How much fun are those kinds of animals that just sit there and chew grass in a tiny, smelly cage? I don't know any of my friends who got particularly involved with their animals.

I can somewhat understand the joy of having a dog, though. It understands what you're saying and shows up when you want it to. It can also be good for exercise or companionship, from what I understand. But a dog would really inconvenience us and, as I said, I don't like animals. I have noticed that it's best to keep quiet about not liking animals. If you tell people, they look down on you and think that you're an empathically disturbed person. You sort of have to think animals are sweet, cuddly, and helpless creatures that need to be taken care of. It may be the case that someone needs to take care of them, but it's not going to be me. I will say that I actually think they are really disgusting. They eat strange things, lick their butts, bite even though you haven't done anything, have long, dirty claws that need to be cut, and are generally unreliable. Add the enormous costs for food, insurance, veterinary care, and wine bottles and chocolate for the pet sitter during vacations, and it adds up to the cost of a family trip to a warm climate . . . per year.

With that starting point in mind, you get a better picture of how much work my kids put into trying to convince me to buy an animal. Since I'm not an empathically disturbed person, their nagging or, more correctly, pleas, didn't leave me completely unmoved. I saw and heard their yearning and I knew that my children were smart, so I felt like I needed to listen to them. However, listening is one thing and doing something they want you to do is another, I know that. When this whole animal thing was brought up for the first time, Sara was five and Daniel was three. Sara's best friend had gotten a hamster and Sara was there almost every day to pet it. The friend's parents told us how convenient the little hamster was: "They're very easy to take care of, the cage only needs to be cleaned once a week, and they only need a little food and water." Although it's a nocturnal animal and it runs a little on its wheel at night, we just move the cage into the laundry room. They also only live for a few years.

Yes, that's nice, I thought—planning the burial when you've only just bought the little creature. Sara had a long list of arguments that she shared with her mother Lena and me. I argued politely and logically explaining nocturnal animals weren't much fun, as they needed to sleep during the day and it would be a pain to clean the cage every week, and that they only lived for two years. "So, what about a raaaabbit?"

This is the way it continued and I had to admire the children for their persistence. As they kept pressing, and got their little brother involved, I started to feel a little bad. Lena changed her opinion and became more and more inclined to think that "a small animal might be nice and even a good thing for the kids." Why am I so stubborn, and isn't my word the law in this family? No, I don't like animals and my children don't like to sail on our boat, which is my favorite thing to do, yet they have always had to come along on the weekends.

In the end, something occurred to me. I don't think it was my guilty conscience, perhaps more of an insight. The kids had played fair all along and I thought that I had listened to them, but . . . I don't think that I actually heard them out. I raised the subject with Lena when it was just the two of us and she found that I had a point in my reasoning, although she felt that I was a little hard on myself. You're a good dad, but I know you don't like animals—maybe you can get used to it? That was the moment when I started thinking about it from a different point of view. Could I get used to animals?

I took it as a sign when I came home from work a few days later and the neighbor's cat, Lola, showed up and rubbed against my leg. It was almost a bit spooky! That cat had never cared about me. Could it be feeling that I had softened up and was turning into an animal lover? As I calmed down, I came up with a brilliant idea. The neighbor wasn't very interested in her cat. She would hardly notice if we borrowed it for a day. It was always running around outside, even at night. I suggested my idea to Lena who thought I was totally crazy but admitted that it was one really fun idea. We talked a lot about how we would present this to the children. We didn't want them to think that it was okay to just take an animal when you felt like it (though that was exactly what we were going to do, or borrowing it, actually). What if they couldn't keep our secret and accidentally said something?

Lena and I thought it was so funny, so we decided to do it. We told Daniel and Sara that we were going to borrow Lola next weekend. "Is the neighbor letting us do that?" asked the children. We had prepared ourselves for that question and made up that it was a surprise for Lola. We would take care of her as if she were a princess cat. We would give her lots of nice food and we would pet her all the time and it would be our's and Lola's secret. Secrets always appeal to kids. They were very happy and started to plan Lola's "luxury weekend."

The following Friday we bought really fancy cat food—the sticky kind in a jar, a bag of dry food, and some shrimp. We had agreed on a luxury weekend and we would have one! I had even bought kitty litter that we filled a shoebox with. When the weekend arrived, the kids got to stay up a little later and I snuck out at dusk (Lena refused to) with some fresh shrimp as bait. I had the guts to make some *ksssss ksssss* noises as well. Lola often sat on our neighbor's stairs and that's where I found her. She came right away, I didn't even have to reveal the shrimp and it wasn't difficult to take her home to our house after that. Luckily, our house blocks the view from the neighbor's side. I pondered a little about whether anyone had seen me, but I decided to just ignore it. Being nice to a cat must be allowed!

And then Lola's luxury weekend started. We gave her a lot of goodies and she was showered with petting and snuggles. The kids were thrilled, Lena and I felt mischievous, and I personally felt like a cool dad, who had organized a cat for the kids. I can't say that I fell in love with animals just because I had come up with such a good idea, but it was actually a lot of fun and Lola was really friendly for a cat. Above all, it was nice seeing how good the kids were with the cat. Lola got to stay the night, as I had promised, and she was "ours" the whole Saturday. She must have thought she was in heaven! As Saturday evening arrived, Lola started to circle around the front door and our cat toilet had only been used once, so we knew it was time to let her out.

Then what happened?

It was cool having a secret with the neighbor's cat. The children have never mentioned it to her, from what I know. In retrospect, I don't think she would have minded us borrowing Lola, but it wouldn't have been as much fun. The children were excited but we felt like a cat would be too much of a responsibility. I agreed to getting a bunny after some persuasion. I promised that I would try to learn to like bunnies and our Bruno in particular. However, I would not have to take care of it if I didn't want to.

Having Bruno works well and the kids really take care of him with some help from Lena and myself. I don't love Bruno and we don't really understand each other, but he lives here, and so do I, and in some way, we both accept this. It's different with Lola; we usually have a talk when I get home from work, reminiscing about our secret, and we've talked about doing the luxury weekend again.

New thoughts

I need to be more open to things that at first seem intolerable. Above all, I need to listen more. Listening doesn't necessarily mean agreeing, I don't think anyone else has thought this either. Lola is good. It can be a good idea borrowing an animal to try it out and get used to it for a bit. Common secrets bring families closer and give us something fun to remember.

Walk the limit

I've clearly explained to my son where he isn't allowed to play and now I'm stuck in the Land of Limits and Nos. Help me get out of here!

Steven with Nora, age 4, and Emile, age 7.

When Emile was two years old, we moved from an apartment to a townhouse. Living in a townhouse wasn't our biggest dream, but it was what we could afford if we wanted to live close to a big city. We liked it from the beginning—the nearby forest and the park and large grassy areas where we felt safe letting our young child play.

We wanted our children to be able to roam quite freely, obviously depending on their age and maturity, but we wanted them to get out easily. We had a romantic image of living in a real house painted by two people raised in apartments, but we still have that idyllic feeling; it's cozy living in a townhouse with all the kids in the yard and all the neighbors who go out as soon as the sun comes out.

There are a lot of families living in the neighborhood and there are loads of kids in the area in the early summer. They play soccer, ride on their bikes, and do all the things that children have done throughout history. It's especially cool when various games are organized, such as kick the can or hide and seek with lots of kids of all ages. Everyone is welcome to join and there's a great courtyard community where everyone has fun.

When Emile was younger, we kept a constant eye on him, who he visited, where he went. He was also quite happy with the limits on where he could go. But the older he got, the more space he wanted, so he disappeared quite often. All of a sudden he was gone and a slight unease immediately appeared in his father or mother's stomach. Where is the kid?

We would look everywhere, scream across the yard, check with the neighbors, and finally, when we expected the worst possible scenario, he showed up completely unaware and indifferent to our questions and worried hugs. He'd just been playing.

There is also a large common space near our neighborhood with some rocks and a small forest, which is perfect for building huts and adventures, so this was naturally the place he usually went.

"You can't go to the forest by yourself!"

"You shouldn't go anywhere without asking!"

"You have to bring Mom or Dad!"

"We get worried when we can't find you and you don't hear us calling."

In the end, all the musts and warnings were too much for Emile, so he lost it and shouted at me: "What can I do? You just say 'can't' and 'don't' all the time? What caaan I do?"

Well, what can you do when you are five? How far beyond the yard are you allowed to go? Which friends can you visit? What can five-year-old Emile really do? I had to think about what I would allow him to do. I pondered and visited one of our neighbors, a mother who also had a five-year-old and asked her the same question, "What's Anthony allowed to do? How far can he wander off?"

This mother agreed with my reasoning and ideas. We decided fairly quickly on a lot of "gets," and made a whole list of them.

You get to visit a friend if you tell us that you're going there.

You get to ride the bike in the yard if you're wearing a helmet.

You're get to hang out anywhere in the territory for five-year-olds if you tell someone that you're leaving.

This was a risk on our part because we needed Emile's and Anthony's advice on how big the territory they could stay in should be. We were only parents, how could we know exactly what the border would look like?

The following day we brought the boys out to decide what the territory for the five-year-olds was going to be. We told them that there was a limit to how far a five-year-old could go and because they both were at the right age, they knew best what was too far. This is how "walk the limit" started; we walked along the area and the boys continuously conferred with each other and with us.

"The hill, are we allowed to be on the hill?"

"Yes, the little one," I thought.

"Hmm, but not on the other side because then you won't hear when our fathers are calling," said Emile, remembering our last fight.

We strode on and after a while the five-year-old limit became visible for us and for them. What was interesting was that their limit was fine, I hadn't interfered, but I thought that their limits were very similar to mine.

"Well," said Anthony's mother, "shall we walk around your five-year-old territory?"

We strode on in single file and the boys were very proud and happy with themselves; they had single-handedly decided on the border and we had only to follow. As a consequence, there were more kids in the neighborhood that joined our five-year-old limit and Emile and Anthony were always keen to walk around the territory to show it to the new five-year-olds.

Then what happened?

We have come up with a six-year-old limit and seven-year-old limit, to meet the demand.

We create the border together and the territory expands a little each year. We now have a limit to how far they're allowed to ride their bikes without being accompanied by an adult. It's like a fence that expands a little each year and you're allowed to move quite freely inside it. The borders are ignored from time to time and sometimes the odd mistake occurs, but that's natural, who wouldn't want to check whether the fencing is up to standard?

New thoughts

Our children are incredibly competent and fun to work with; we did this together and the biggest lesson that I learned was very much about what I win by being positive and open-minded instead of negative and forbidding.

The fact that we could mutually decide and come to an agreement that we both felt comfortable with has helped me to trust Emile more, and he feels that his voice matters when we need to enforce boundaries. Me listening to him is fundamental for us being able to agree.

The monster trap

Lucas started having more nightmares and with the nightmares came worries about falling asleep and waking up in the middle of the night. Despite our promises that there wasn't a monster living under his bed or in the closet, he knew. The monster was there.

Anna with Lucas, age 6, Julie, age 10, and Marcus, age 13.

Now and then, Lucas went through long periods when he would have nightmares and restless sleep, which affected the whole family. This usually happened during difficult transitions in his life, like when we moved him to a new daycare or his best friend moved. Incidents that forced him to rearrange his thinking and process new events and thoughts. He is a thinker and he doesn't tell us everything, so his mind obviously became full of various ideas and impressions. The older children had never had nightmares or any problems sleeping, they could fall asleep with a lamp lit and sleep like a stone, so this was a new challenge for us. He would sometimes wake up and just cry, calling out for one of us, and we had to come as quickly as firemen, or he would become completely hysterical. He was too scared to go to our room because you never knew what or who would catch him on the way to our bedroom.

This was about life and death for him and it was really difficult for us. When we talked to him about the night monsters during the day he would listen, agreeing that there wasn't anything under the bed, he went through the closet with us, so he intellectually understood exactly what we were trying to explain, but when darkness fell, it was a different story.

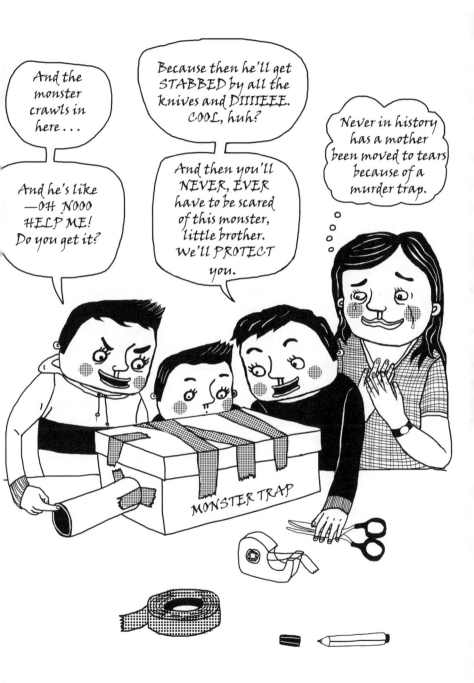

Lamps needed to be lit, we would check under the bed and in boxes together, and when that procedure was completed, he would lie there there tensely and couldn't sleep. Windows were rustling and he heard murmuring underneath the bed. Each time this happened, we immediately had to be at his assistance before the monster would show up. The whole family was finally involved in this monster hunt, his brothers searched, we supported him, and Lucas cried.

His older brother, Marcus, finally found a solution: If you can't beat them, join them! He and Lucas built a cool giant monster trap. They duct taped a large shoebox, cut a hole, and stuck a paper towel tube in it, and on the inside there were sharp spikes that would make the monster get stuck in the box once he crawled into it. With this long entrance and a chamber with spikes that was impossible to escape, the monster would be stuck. They were both very proud of their design and it had to be tested right away. What bait do you use for monsters? Candy was a great suggestion, especially if his brothers got some money to buy it and the monster hunters got the leftovers.

The trap was set and placed in a strategic space in the closet, far from Lucas's bed. A row of candies stretched before the tube entrance. What monster could resist jelly beans and gummy bears? At the far end of the trap a small bowl of detergent was placed, because monsters are allergic to it and die immediately if they come into contact with it. Marcus told Lucas that if a monster was killed in the trap, the detergent would turn into water and then you could just pour it out in the toilet and it was gone. We were with them all the way, because nothing we tried earlier had cured his fears, so this was perhaps the best way to affirm his monster and help him defeat it. Some nights we would swap detergent for water when he had fallen asleep and when he discovered it, he got to pour the monster down the toilet. He would walk around with the bowl and make sure that the whole family saw what he had accomplished, and he was proud as a peacock. After that, we began to pour the water less frequently—there were hardly any monsters left, indeed—extinction was close. He would still wake up at night, but he wasn't as heart-wrenchingly terrified. One of us would at times have to crawl into the closet and check on the trap, but when we found it was empty, he calmed down.

Then what happened?

We are having a quiet period at the moment. Lucas is in an incredibly happy mood. He feels comfortable with himself, with us, with his new preschool. There is very little talk of monsters; we check the trap from time to time, but we never catch anything. He also sleeps much better; he wakes up sometimes and will come to us on his own and crawl in, so we don't have to get him anymore. We had a lot of fun playing monster hunting together and the best part was that his big brothers were so committed to making their little brother's life easier. We were just like a team that would scare away the night monster together. They've never teased Lucas about his fears, but they still tease him about everything else when the opportunity arises.

New thoughts

I like the idea of being in the worlds of my children, to feel what they feel. It's good to fantasize about things together so they become real. Not everything must be done in my adult, rational, and realistic way; there are big benefits in me daring to be childish. We beat the monster! Others think we're a little crazy, but at the same time, who decides what can exist and cannot exist? Santa Claus and the tooth fairy are accepted, so why not a monster or a ghost? Sooner or later, reality crawls up on you and the truth, our truth, is revealed. Santa Claus doesn't exist!

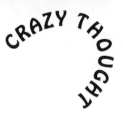

Dinner guests

I have lost my will and can't be bothered to cook. My inspiration is more dead than the sausage I finally throw onto the table.

Peter with Brian, age 5, and Bobby, age 6.

Planning meals is so boring. Every day is a struggle to come up with new ideas. We've ended up in a rut of spaghetti and meatballs. Sometimes we go out on a limb and make pancakes with fruit and cream. Meals should be quick to make and nutritious, filling, and preferably edible for the kids. I enjoy cooking food and finding new recipes and trying out exciting flavors, but this only happens when I have the time and energy, which is usually during the weekend. I don't know what to cook Monday through Friday. Camilla and I usually have a greasy lunch at a restaurant and don't feel like making real food for dinner. We could settle for soup or a hot sandwich, but the kids obviously have to get fed. This is the way it turns out: We come home late, open all the cabinets, and find nothing to cook. This happens far too often. No one has gone grocery shopping because we both think that the other one did. Or we simply forget. Look in the freezer and find frozen meatballs or a dull old package of bacon. Pasta topped with fish sticks and sweet corn was one of those "we're out of everything" dinners.

I'll feel paralyzed and don't even want to enter the kitchen and begin. Zero inspiration and zero passion for food. But the kids are pretty happy regardless of what we put out on the table, in my opinion they have a fairly simple taste of what tastes good, so almost anything will do.

For a period of time we always had at least one extra kid for dinner who happily ate whatever was on the table. The strategy was the following: A friend of the kids' dropped in and asked if they could play, about an hour before dinnertime. Our kid would wait until dinner was nearly ready and asked if Jason, Kristin, or Lauren could also eat with us. When we'd answer yes they'd call their parents who probably burst with happiness that they wouldn't have to worry about it. Everyone was happy. We knew we'd have a quiet dinner since we had a dinner guest, the kids enjoyed having a friend over, and the other parents had peace of mind and wouldn't even have to worry about making dinner if they weren't hungry. Everyone won. I thought it was great because everyone at the table seemed to appreciate the food more with the outside company. My kids ate more when we had dinner guests than when it was only us eating our usual meatballs.

However, I started thinking whether I should also try the eating-at-a-friend's-house strategy for a while—we always had a dinner guest, surely other parents were willing to do the same. I decided to try it out at least once a week. We lived in an area with many children and Brian and Bobby have many friends, so it would probably work.

Normally, I told them "no" when they wanted to go to someone's house and play before dinner but now I started saying "yes." Off they went and I could eat a sandwich and read the newspaper. After half an hour the phone would ring:

"Can I eat at Kelsie's?"

"That's fine with me, what does Kelsie's mother think?"

"It's fine with her, she says," said my son.

"Okay, you have to be home by 6:30, will you tell her or should I?"

"You can tell her."

Then Kelsie's mother would take the phone and say of course it was fine, we had Kelsie over for dinner so many times.

Yes, it worked!

Then what happened?

From time to time, we have a dinner guest, but the kids eat elsewhere quite often. They think it's great and sometimes I hear them comparing dinners with each other—who made the most delicious meat sauce or who made the best-tasting food. Because of this, they will call ahead and check what food is being served at Kelsie's and if they like our food better, they'll stay home. Picky rascals. We've been trying a new thing with two other families of having a joint dinner every week, so we organize dinner at each other's homes every third Wednesday, and it's been really nice.

We are only on the second round so far, but it's been working out great; tasty food is served, it's exciting eating out, and I go home feeling inspired to find new recipes every time. We enjoy cooking once it's our turn, because it's like having a party, a regular day party!

New thoughts

How I can make everyday food more fun is my biggest concern. How do I get out of a meal planning rut? There should be a television show that helps families find joy in making food every day. I can be the first one to try it; I'll sign up voluntarily.

Another thought is how much fun they have when they eat at their friends' houses, where they can be social and behave in a different way than they would at home. We've seen how friendly and polite our boys are when they are away at dinner, but we don't exactly see much of that.

Packing Mom's suitcase

Packing really sucks! I cringe when I just think of packing. For some reason, which I don't understand, I have become (probably by my own choice) the family packing master. I also get blamed if we forget to bring anything. I dread the process of packing several days before going away, and once I do it, I feel really irritated. Neither I nor anyone else in the family has any fun and all trips start with me being very angry and frustrated while the rest of the family tiptoes around me.

Petra with Nick, age 3, and Alice, age 5.
My idea would be controversial, but I was so tired of packing for the whole family that I made the suggestion before our trip to the grandparents' house for Easter break. A few days before, I dropped the bomb that we should pack for each other—the kids would pack for me and I would pack for the children—and the children were thrilled. Now we got to play! We talked about important things to consider when packing and I suggested the following questions to put on their checklist: How long are we going to be away for? What are we going to be doing? What do I think the weather will be like? What do I want to do indoors and outdoors? How much can I carry? A good trick is to think chronologically, from the time you leave until when you get back and then take things out as you go along. Then you place

everything on the bed and do a final check before putting it in the bag! And you'll have to keep in mind that it's me you're packing for. "Yep, that's the way to deal with them," I thought to myself happily after my course on packing.

Okay, the kids were five and three years old and I could somewhat see that what I said didn't always register with them, but I repressed that. We were having fun! The kids were happy and I was happy. The days leading up to Easter were really nice and we joked about all the crazy things that we could pack: the bed, all the books on the bookshelf, all the toys, the rubber ducks, just candy and no food. "Should we pack the food too?" asked the five-year-old, but I'd reached my limit at that point. To get past it, without spoiling all the fun, I found myself quickly saying that we'd shop on the way (Oh, that was close, imagine an entire Easter weekend in the country with nothing but candy!). The three-year-old doesn't mind leaving his toys and bed and I'm glad that I have a five-year-old, too. I actually tried not to influence them with disguised advice, and it was a real challenge. My mantra was: How bad could it be? I tried to use the question rhetorically and pushed away all the unpleasant answers that crept into my mind.

I'd have to work that Thursday and I decide that we'd pack on Friday morning since we weren't in a hurry (at least it was one less night). The children woke up early on Good Friday and I did too. It was actually going to be great going to the country house. We decide that they'd pack in my room and I'd pack in theirs and that it was forbidden to peek. Alice, who understood what this trip was all about, still couldn't resist talking about how nice it would be when she and Nick got their Easter eggs on Saturday. I get the hint but played stupid.

I packed as usual, but without the thousand questions I usually asked the kids, like do you want to bring this or that, or maybe this? I simply did my best to try to think of what they really wanted to bring, and I thought it was nice and pleasant thinking about what they liked to do and wear. I also tried to pack something that they didn't expect me to pick.

I heard the rattle of hangers, slamming of drawers, giggles, and whispers, and tripping coming from my room. My packing was taking longer than usual, but it was a lot more fun. After an hour, I was done. I sat down on the couch and waited. A while later Nick showed up because he didn't want to pack anymore. I put a movie on for him and cuddled for a while before Alice came in with a happy face and a packed bag. We were very eager to leave because we, especially Alice and I, were so curious to see what the other had packed.

When we arrived, unpacking was like opening Christmas presents. The children were pleased as well as surprised by the contents of their bags. My bag consisted of my nicest clothes and it felt really nice going around the countryside in a shiny light blue dress. They had also managed to pack a book for me. I had in fact already read that particular book, which led to an interesting conversation with the children about why adults want to read their books only once and children about a hundred times. We talked a lot about the packing and what we liked the most and least about it.

Then what happened?

We're looking forward to the next time we travel and pack for each other. This was a fun and great way for everyone to feel responsible for our trip planning. The older Nick gets, the more involved he'll become. In order not to wear out the fun maybe we might not do it every time, but I also think that it teaches the kids how to think when they're packing for themselves.

New thoughts

Much of my packing anxiety has been about my need for control. What I choose to pack for the kids is determined by what I think is practical and what they should bring with them rather than what they actually want to bring.

They haven't been dissatisfied with my packing, but neither are they particularly excited about it. It's amazing what confidence the children have in me as a parent doing things for them. This is more "packing with love" instead of "packing with force," because we make an effort to select things that we think the other person wants to bring.

Are there other bad habits we can fix?

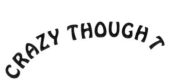

The World Cup of sibling fights

My god, do my kids argue with each other. I don't want to get involved in these fights in any way, but will they kill each other if I go on strike?

Constance with Camilla, age 8, Theresa, age 6, and Simon and Lucas, age 4. I don't have siblings myself (perhaps this is why I chose to have so many children) and thus never had someone to argue with. In my family we never teased one another, or, more accurately, we didn't have loud fights. Sure, we would get angry, but we often sulked and went our separate ways, closing the door behind us. Dealing with things that bothered us wasn't our thing, and it was different for me because I lived with two adults who solved conflicts in a "mature" way. I remember that I often felt angry and that I had arguments and even fights with my friends, as I had to find an outlet for my feelings, and they were as close to siblings as they could be. I was really too old to be fighting and I was also a girl, so when this happened, I was ashamed because I didn't follow the norm. I remember thinking that it was really scary when my friends had arguments with their families in front of me. It was louder and so much more open than in our house.

Over time, I became an expert at arguing. I argued my way out of just about anything, including my grades. No one could win in a fight against me. I think many people found me really annoying. I loved hanging out with guys because my way of being suited theirs better, and I had a really hard time making girlfriends. It wasn't until high school that I started making real girlfriends and it was so incredibly nice to share my life with other girls. It wasn't until that point that I really understood how I should redirect my fierce temper to not hurt others.

During this time, I had several relationships with guys but I didn't have the courage to argue with them, because of my fear of being left. I was twenty years old when I met my future husband, Peter. It was a love that sneaked up on me and I didn't have any plans to be in a long relationship. Eighteen years and four children later, we are still a couple and it feels like we will be one forever. Peter was the one I started fighting with properly. We screamed, erupted, and threw stuff. Both of us were allowed to be angry. No one left and we loved each other, even after the fights were over. Eventually the intensity of our fights faded; today they happen now and then, with the same intensity but with different modes of expression. Still, it feels good to be able to argue with Peter because I know that we can resolve our conflicts and frustrations that way.

I can, therefore, see and understand that my children's fights fulfill a function. They seek out each other when they need to fight, and when I'm wise and really think about it, I understand that they choose to fight with the people they feel most comfortable with. At time, in the heat of the moment, I go mad and wonder what's wrong with my children who fight so much. It's also interesting to observe how the kids fight in different ways. I'm scared to analyze it, but I can imagine that it has to do with their various ages, different personalities, and maybe their gender. Some of my friends tell me about how their daughters argue more verbally than their sons do, who are more physical. As a girl, it's often about getting the last word in, while boys want the last hit.

For a period of time, they were getting into more trouble than usual; there was yelling, hitting, pinching, crying, and fights almost every day. None of the angels were innocent. For a while we called the girls Scream and Panic, one started teasing, the other hit or pinched in defense, the first screamed out loud and chased the person who hit her, preferably with a weapon so that whoever was being chased roared even more. Very charming! We had to physically keep them apart and acted as cop and judge; it was never anyone's fault and it was always the other one who had started it.

The boys wrestled and fought instead, which usually started out like an innocent game, then one of them would get a stronger punch than

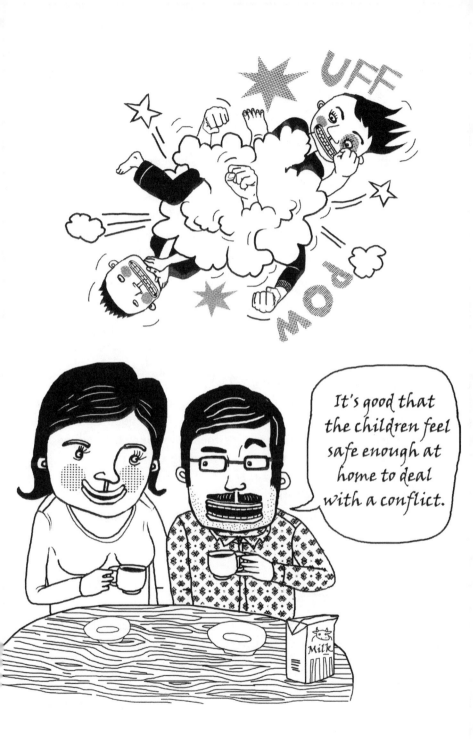

expected and it would take off from there. Fights including tears, yelling, and large chunks of hair flying around. Not very charming either!

I was really fed up with this and Peter and I thought a lot about how to put an end to it. Nothing we had done had worked, so we had to think of new ideas. Peter thought that we should get boxing gloves and let them fight in a knockout round, but I drew the line there.

I bought a notebook and wrote a list of a hundred different things the family could do. It was fun stuff, like tickling a sibling or getting a soda in the middle of the week; easy things like going out for ice cream, and chores like helping to fold laundry or wash dishes, but all of them were there to divert fights. Every time there was trouble in the air, we brought out the list. Whoever had fought had to pick a number; sometimes you would be lucky and other times you'd be unlucky. But it was something to talk about and it was fun and exciting.

After that list was done, the four of them printed out drawings of legless spiders on the computer. The deal was that every time someone walked away from a fight between others without joining in, he would draw one leg on a spider and when the spider had all eight legs, you got to do something fun with Mom or Dad. This bribe-and-divert system worked pretty well for a while, and then everyone began to brag to each other, who had and who hadn't done what. It was good because the fights ended pretty quickly, but now there was more tattletaling and stabbing in the back. We also tried a running competition which we really enjoyed; whoever was arguing had to get dressed and run around our neighborhood and the person who won the race had won the fight. Everyone agreed on it in the beginning, but that competition didn't work in the long run either. Because how do you force someone to run if they sit down and refuse?

Then what happened?

Sure, they continue to fight! It comes and goes in periods. Sometimes it's as quiet as ever and we think we have the sweetest and nicest kids in the world, but that can change within an hour and chaos and panic reappear.

The boys are getting along at the moment, so they tease their sisters instead, who in turn gossip and whine, and it's almost worse than the fights. I get so sick of it. Regardless of how and why the kids fight, I think that they need to continue doing it. My theory, that fighting is a way to get rid of frustration, sadness, and anger, isn't really accurate, because many times I think it's about getting attention from us adults or from siblings. See me, love me.

No matter how difficult I think it is when they are arguing, I can still say that fighting can actually be healthy for a family; everyone can be themselves and feel safe.

New thoughts

I can't divert everything, they have to deal with some of the drama themselves. Whatever I do to try to end the fight, it's going to continue. Sometimes I have to deal with the situation and accept that sibling fights are a part of being a family. It's actually often my own problem, because I suffer the most from all the fights; the others usually seem quite happy with the family's "level of fighting."

I need to find a balance that works for me; all the fights won't end just because I want them to. We have yet to see the winner of the The World Cup of sibling fights.

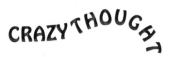

CRAZY THOUGHT

We're so good at lying

Others try to plan our family weekends, holidays, and vacations. Dinner parties and visits feel like forced obligations. Telling the truth is bitter and I'm afraid of hurting others.

Eva with Leo, age 2, and Holly, age 4.
When Holly was born, she was the first grandchild on both sides and the expectant grandmothers had prepared big time for this long-awaited little girl. The fight over who would be the most important grandmother started before she was born. Each time we came back from the obstetrician, my mother and mother-in-law would call to make sure that the baby was growing the way it should, that I was feeling well and taking care of myself, and they wanted to know exactly what the doctor had said, and what Stephen thought.

It was good but also disturbing that there was such a huge interest in something that was so important in our lives, but I also felt obliged to report every single change and occurrence.

Both Stephen I and had cut the umbilical cord to our parents and we had a very simple and straightforward relationship with them. We are adults, we do what we want, and we do what we do. They had the right to think and have opinions, but it was our life. That attitude worked for us, up until we announced that we were going to have children.

I couldn't tell you what day it was when I realized that this wouldn't be smooth sailing, but it happened sometime in the middle of my first pregnancy. A power struggle started to form between the two families, which came in the form of wishing us the best, in order to get as much as possible for themselves.

Mother-in-law: "You have to come over this weekend so that I can pamper you before the baby comes. You need to rest and take it easy, because there won't be any time for that later."

My mother: "Will you come by before the baby comes? No? Why? You're going over there, but we don't get to take care of you. Then you'll have to come to our place first when the baby has arrived."

This is the way it went on. One of them would remind us of family names on one side of the family and the other one told us that if it were a boy, his middle name would have to be Theodore.

We probably didn't realize what we had started. We tried to be as passive as possible for the longest time and make everyone happy. When I went into labor, we were stupid enough to call them both and tell them that it was happening. It was our first child so we didn't know any better; we probably had an image in our heads that we would be done in a few hours and that we would call and tell them the news after that. The delivery ward probably never had received that many calls from expecting grandmothers as they did that day. We just wanted to be left alone, but eventually Stephen had to phone them and tell them that they had to stop calling because they were bothering us and that we didn't have the time or the desire to update their curious minds every hour. We've subsequently had to pay for this. That's one of the few times when they've actually agreed—that was no way to treat a worried expectant grandmother.

They both wanted to pay for the baby stroller, and they ended up splitting it between them, to make it fair. They turned into two children and they were blind to what we wanted or felt. It was a really a screwed-up situation. But at the same time, their commitment to our children was quite amazing. They loved our kids and we never had a problem with getting them to babysit or help out. It was almost as if they would give their lives up to be there for us. From talking to friends, I've understood that the position we were in is worth millions, especially since there are a lot of people who don't have anyone to ask for help.

I don't know when we started lying, but all of these concerns were suffocating us:

Whose weekend was it to get the grandson?

Where would we celebrate Christmas?

Who would we visit during our vacation?

Who would come over during the weekend?

Where would we have Sunday dinner?

Everything, absolutely everything, was a struggle for justice and we felt like we were being pushed into a corner.

Stephen and I tried to talk to our parents a number of times, to get them to understand that we needed a little refreshing indifference. But this didn't work, as they both had become completely blind, according to us, anyway.

So we started lying.

It started out with fairly small innocent lies about us having a stomach virus and that there was no point in coming over for Sunday dinner. But perhaps another Sunday?

Then we were at Stephen's parents' house, and they asked us to come with them out to the country for Easter. I felt my whole body saying no and then I heard Stephen say:

"No, we can't. We've already promised some old friends of Eva's that we're going down to see them. How did you know them again, Eva? Was it an old classmate?"

So I elaborated, not too much, but just enough to make it sound believable. It was as easy as ever. We made it a habit. I would lie to my parents about us meeting Stephen's friends and he lied to his. We knew the truth—that we wanted time alone—would hurt, so we went with the lies. So far we've made up that we drove cross-country, been to a lot of different places, met quite a few invisible friends during these years, and we've even attended a made-up wedding. We've had a lot of fun and helped each other out with our lies. It wasn't pretty, but it worked.

Then what happened?

The older Holly gets, the more difficult the lying gets, because we don't want our children to become liars, not even for a good cause.

Holly is four years old now and very aware of what we say and don't say and corrects us if we do something wrong, so we have adjusted our lies to this, too. The era of big lies is over and now it's time for the little white lies.

The grandmothers have also calmed down a little, but they are really important for the kids and for us, too. We don't want to disagree with them, but we are the ones who decide how we want things in our family. We're not going to let others dictate the terms for visits or how to spend our time.

We have also become better at setting limits and speaking up about when we can't or don't want to do something, without having to come up with long explanations, excuses, or insane lies.

New thoughts

No, not really. I'm a little ashamed about all this lying, but it's been pretty fun at the same time. In addition, what we have gained has been great and as far as I know, we haven't hurt anyone.

Stephen and I have enjoyed ourselves and created shared stories that we have been able to laugh heartily at. At times it gets a little crazy, especially when we have forgotten to tell the other person that we told a lie and you have to stand there keeping a straight face; this is when a good poker face comes in handy.

Sleeping on the couch

I'm tired of our never-ending nighttime walks between the bedroom and living room. The carpet is almost worn out. We are a mother and a father who sit on the couch watching television like two ragdolls and unwillingly take turns leading or carrying two little rascals back and forth, who can't or won't sleep.

Mia with Niels, age 5, and Melvin, age 6.

Last spring we had hellish nights, not occasionally, but every single night. It all worked fine except for the actual sleeping. We haven't thought much about our routines that we've had since the boys were really young; it always just worked. They'd get an evening snack, a shower or bath, brushed their teeth, get a bedtime story, and then they slept. But suddenly, the boys became restless. After a last kiss and when it was time to calm down, it all started.

The door to the boys' room had to be open a precise number of inches, the bathroom door next to them had to be open and have the lights on, while the door to the living room had to be open so that they could hear the TV. That was the simple list of rules that was communicated every night. After everything was done according to their instructions, one of them would always get up to open the door the tiniest bit. Then, someone would always think their bed was itchy, so we had to brush off invisible crumbs, smooth out the microscopic crinkles of the blankets, and run around like housekeepers getting water, fluffing pillows, and giving extra hugs. When we reached this point of our marathon service, Jon or I became the angry police who yelled and shouted. This made one or both of them sad and they needed comforting and talking to before they could stop crying. After this, we usually collapsed on the couch like two tired pillows and this was when the tiptoeing began.

Tip, tap, tip. "I can't sleep!"

"Go to bed!"

"It's too dark!" "It's too hot!" "I want another pillow!"

It was back and forth every evening; if it wasn't one thing, it was another. Our evenings were full of crying, yelling, and there was generally a bad atmosphere. We were very exhausted after a long day of work and that moment in the evening, when the boys had gone to bed, was our only time to relax. We needed it so much and never got it.

One evening when Jon was doing something for work and I was alone with the boys, I felt that I couldn't run the evening circus by myself, so I made the couch up for the three of us to lie in. After brushing our teeth, we cuddled on the cushions, with the teddy bears and blankets. The boys lay next to each other and I lay head to feet with them. We chatted for a while, they liked lying on the couch and being with me. I half-watched TV while lying there and then the first kid fell asleep and then the other one gave up and shut his eyes. I felt that the concept was working well, but I felt that it was more about the novelty, and eventually, they would go back to their usual nighttime rituals. But Jon wanted to continue sleeping on the couch and also took it a step further by letting the boys choose where they wanted to sleep—on the cozy couch with Mom and Dad, or in their own beds. The couch was the obvious choice for a period of time, but then Melvin wanted to sleep in his own bed and we didn't make a big deal of it. The choice was theirs. Our evenings were a lot quieter and if one of us didn't want to lie on the couch with the whole group, we would take turns. We weren't tired as much, and maintained a better mood.

Then what happened?

It's been a year and I can't really grasp what was so difficult. I remember the feelings and all the fights, but I don't understand how we ended up in that mess. Now it feels like we made a really big deal out of something quite small. Both of us also worked a lot during that period of time, and the boys felt that they didn't get the attention that they needed, and they expressed that by trying to get as much of us as possible while they were awake, or at least something along those lines. Everything surrounding the sleeping procedure has become so much easier, perhaps because we make everything a lot easier. We are no longer stuck in our routines, which I still think are good, but we've become more flexible. The boys will still fall asleep on the couch at times, other times they fall asleep in our bed, sometimes in their own, and the hardest part for me is getting them into their own beds when they fell asleep in ours, I feel like it strains my back. In a year, I probably won't be able to lift them anymore.

New thoughts

I want to spend time with my boys; they're smart and they clearly express when they feel they didn't get enough time with me by causing fights in the evening. That's my interpretation of it anyway. Another thing I've been thinking of concerning sleeping routines is that it's really important and time saving to have a routine, but when it doesn't work, what is it that makes you wait so long to change it? Trying something new doesn't mean that it will be that way forever, but if I don't try it, I won't know if it will work or not. I think Jon and I were so tired and drained at that point that we didn't see any opportunities, but just continued with our habitual rut.

Trading places

I want to be little, I want to be a child, be pampered, dressed, and served breakfast. The ultimate reward would be a baby carriage big enough for an adult, where I could be tucked in and rest, while someone pushed me to work.

Abigail with Talia, age 6, and Jay, age 9.
I am alone with the children full-time for about nine months out of the year because their dad works abroad and is only home occasionally. It works well for the most part, but it can be quite tiresome at times. Our routines and habits contribute to making our everyday life relatively painless. But sometimes we all end up whining, especially in the mornings. I nag about tooth-brushing, eating breakfast slowly, and other important morning things. Jay is looking for things he misplaced, complaining about schoolbooks, gym clothes, and where is my favorite hat? Talia is yelling and screaming about the wrong choice of clothing, wearing a dress for school and glitter in her hair—she's in a very glamorous phase at the moment. Sometimes I know what kind of morning it's going to be before I leave my bed and I wish I had a butler or nanny who could get the kids organized for me, while I sit and drink my freshly squeezed juice and get my hair done. What a dream! After having a really crappy morning, I decide to become a kid myself. Talia and I nearly had a fight in the hallway over what jacket the glamorous princess would wear and eventually I threw myself down beside my screaming daughter and just lay there. I said nothing, just lay there and looked up, and after a while Hilda said in an adult voice: "We really need to pull ourselves together, Mom. This won't do!"

And so we got up and went on with it. She continued doing her stuff and I got back to mine. But that moment in the hall gave me an idea: I wanted to switch roles; I wanted to be a child in the morning. At dinner the same day I presented my proposal: they would get to be parents the next morning and decide everything; the only important thing was that we had to arrive to school on time. Both of them thought that it was a great and fun game—they would get to decide the whole morning and have their say over me. Talia was even going to take care of the clock radio and the morning alarm. I set my alarm half an hour earlier than usual because I assumed the experiment would take time. Talia was as happy as a clam about organizing the morning schedule. On a normal day, I would have to drag her out of bed after trying to wake her up for five times, but that morning, it was my turn to sleep in. I heard the alarm ring but I pretended to sleep comfortably. I heard the quiet steps across the floor and someone peeing, then quick steps back into the room and boxes going in and out; she was getting dressed, yes! I pretended to be asleep and heard her waking up her brother, who giggled; it felt like someone's birthday or Christmas Eve. I stayed in bed and the door opened.

"It's time to get up, Mom."

"I don't want to, I'm tired," I said in my whiniest voice.

"You have to," said Jay, "or else we'll be late."

"Get up, stupid kid," said Talia.

"Make breakfast and I'll get up," I said. "I want coffee and a sandwich."

"No, you won't have that for breakfast," said the children, "because it's unhealthy, the whining mom is having yogurt and granola."

"Get your clothes on while we make breakfast," Jay called out.

I snuck into the living room half-dressed in my underwear and a T-shirt and that was where they found me in front of the TV, as they appeared with my breakfast. The situation turned serious, I got yelled at for not getting dressed and Talia picked up a pair of ugly socks that she put on me.

"I don't want those socks, they're very ugly," I said and pointed at my feet.

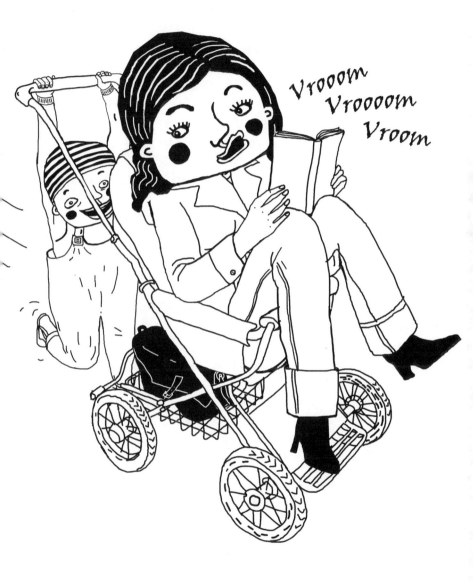

"Now you just shut up and eat," said Talia.

It wasn't pleasant hearing your own voice and words from your six-year-old daughter's mouth. Everything went well—Jay nagged about me eating slowly and Talia had prepared my toothbrush and put it next to me. Things were being rushed.

"It's best that I help you with the brushing because I know how forgetful you usually are," she said.

They were ready in a grown-up way and were just waiting for their infant mom to get ready; they sighed and looked at each other. Wearing no makeup, because that was the rule, even though Tilda curiously checked for mascara, and with clothes chosen by the children, we went to the hallway.

"You have to wear rain boots," said Talia and stared straight at me.

"No, I don't," I said.

"You have to," said Talia and Jay, "it's very wet outside and you can't wear your nice boots today."

"But I can't go to work wearing green rain boots."

"Don't make a fuss now, we are in a hurry, put the boots on. We don't have time for this."

This altercation felt very familiar. It was difficult having to hear your own words again. I felt angry, frustrated, and sweaty, but the children agreed that the rain boots were going on.

"I don't want to play anymore," I said in a squeaky voice. "I want to be an adult now."

"Get a grip, you're not going anywhere in your nice boots" said Jay.

I went to work wearing a coat and rain boots—the children thought that it was necessary due to the weather—but I had to bring my other shoes to wear indoors. Thanks, kids.

Then what happened?

We've done this a couple of times but it was never as good as the first time. It was so serious and earnest the first time, but also fun. I heard myself and my words coming from my children and now I understand how hard it is to be forced into wearing the wrong jacket or ugly boots;

having someone constantly nagging you until you get blisters in your ears. Sure, I still turn into the morning boss when things are moving too slowly, but I probably let the kids take more responsibility for their mornings. They take more responsibility when they get more responsibility, I've always laughed at that and thought that it was a real cliché, but it's actually true.

New thoughts

I'm a kinder mother when I let go of my need for control. The funny part is that before we tried this out, I never thought that my need for control over the kids was that important. But when I let go of the responsibility of feeding them and checking on their clothes, there was suddenly strength and energy left over for other things. At least in the mornings!

Afterword

If we had our way, *Do This! Not That!* would have been as thick as the Bible, but that isn't how the publishing world works. But we can't resist giving you some of the unconventional solutions that we heard from parents that didn't make it in the book. They are in a somewhat random order, but they're really good.

When the child doesn't want to get dressed . . .
- Put your clothes on inside out.
- Put your clothes on blindfolded.
- You choose for the child and the child chooses for you.

When the child doesn't want to go to kindergarten . . .
- Walk backwards to kindergarten.
- Count the steps to kindergarten.
- Find a new way every day.
- Take a random bus and get off at a stop, even if it's heading in the wrong direction.
- Count all the dogs on the way. If you see two, you get an ice cream in the afternoon.

When you just can't be bothered cooking . . .
- Make a weekly menu and use it for as many weeks as you want.
- Only cook TV dinners.
- Make sure that the children are eating plenty of fruits and vegetables . . . in kindergarten and other places.
- Swap menus with other parents.
- Team up with a few parents and make a giant load of food together and then distribute it among everyone.
- Get takeout.

- Play the "sharing game" with the child who won't eat—we'll eat this spoonful, you eat the next one, we'll take this one, you take the next one . . . and so on. Eventually, the plate will be empty. It works best with soup.
- Have dinner without utensils, everyone eats from the same bowls; can be messy but fun.
- Buy a cooking magazine and start cooking from page one, one recipe per day.
- Eat using toothpicks. It's fun to eat potatoes and meatballs by picking them up yourself.
- Arrange dinner outdoors even if it's the middle of winter.

When your child is sick . . .
- Use the "sick bell," a small bell that the sick child can use whenever they need service.
- Use bribes for taking the medicine—all methods are allowed.
- Play rock-paper-scissors in the morning to determine who stays home with the children. Best of three wins.
- The parent who feels like a loser, regardless of whether they go to work or stay at home, gets a surprise from the other person.
- Tell yourself that you don't actually need to be good and do a lot of things, just because you're at home taking care of a sick child. It means being free from responsibility!

When the baby isn't sleeping . . .
- Share the responsibility by including exercise. While one parent sleeps, the other can do bicep curls or squats with the baby.
- Listen to a book on tape while getting a baby to fall asleep.
- Get a nighttime babysitter for a few hours occasionally.

When you have a guilty conscience . . .
- Speak loudly to yourself: I'm doing my best, my child is doing well, I give my child what he/she needs, I take care of the essentials . . .

- Ask yourself the questions: What obligations do I have? Obligations for whom? What do I want?
- Do exactly what your gut tells you.
- Forgive yourself.

When you can't be bothered/don't want to play . . .
- Don't do it!
- Put a movie or a computer game on.
- Make it clear that you don't want to.
- Find someone else who wants to.
- Pay an older sibling to do it.
- Reward yourself when you do it despite not wanting to!

When life is standing still . . .
- Make a change in traditions. Celebrate Christmas and holidays differently than you usually would. Make new traditions for birthdays, etc.
- Do something really exciting that will give you butterflies in the stomach.
- Get something that you can long for, something really fun to think about.
- Do something simple. Rent a movie, call a friend, read a magazine . . .
- Eat something delicious. Chocolate, cheese, mango . . .
- Consider the benefits of something standing still.
- Daydream.

When you're completely exhausted . . .
Ask for help! There are lots of people who can help: neighbors, friends, parents from kindergarten, children's friends' siblings, your siblings . . . Sure, they probably have a lot going on too, but they might not be worn out at the moment. You would surely do the same and help others if they asked you to.

Devote yourself exclusively to the necessary obligations. Ignore the rest or make someone else do it.

We know that there are many people out there that are holding back a lot of cool solutions to everyday problems. To continue with our mission, we need you and your ideas. We are grateful for your parenting stories, but also unique solutions for other areas of life.

You can reach us at our website *www.tvartemot.se,* or visit our Facebook page "The Ultimate Page of Counterintuitive Parenting - Do This Not That."

Please help us to spread the word. Do this by doing the opposite and share it. Be open to talk about the difficult, hard, tedious, and boring, but also the easy and fun things in life as a parent. Gather parents around you and share stories, crazy thoughts, and crazy things you do. You'll get so many ideas and you'll be acknowledged as smart and creative parents. You deserve it!

As a last contribution from us (for now) we give you some wonderful words of advice from Carro's uncle:

"One should spoil their children as much as they can—no more." Think about it and enjoy!

Thank you

We want to say a big thank you to all those who in one way or another contributed to making *Do This! Not That!* happen.

Thank you to all the cool parents who did things differently and who had the courage to share it with us. Thank you to everyone who has shared their difficulties and stood up for their right to both succeed and fail. Oh, how we have laughed (sorry) and cried at all the crazy things you've done.

During the production of this book we have, once again, discovered why we chose to work with parents specifically. What a brave, strong, and creative species! Love and respect!

Thank you to our wonderful families who have coped with us trying out our crazy ideas on them—well, for putting up with us in general. Thank you, beloved Peter and Anders, for dealing with it all, while we sat on a balcony—with a sea view—in Turkey, completing the last parts. We salute all our children and we haven't forgotten about anyone, for being there, keeping us grounded, and making us laugh.

Thank you for reminding us of our own standards and prejudices. It will be of great benefit.

Thank you, Per at Nordstedts for understanding the greatness of *Do This! Not That!* from the first phone call, and believing in our idea and us.

Thank you to all the parents who we had our eye on, and who were the inspiration for many of our ideas—without even knowing it.

Thank you to Ann Ljungberg for priceless advice with everything in terms of marketing and writing—you are professional, as well as resourceful, and truly unconventional.

Last, but not least—a big thanks to the wonderfully funny and talented Lotta Sjöberg who illustrated *Do This! Not That!* and made it perfect and much better than we ever thought it would be.

Åse & Anna